Dr. Liz's

EASY GUIDE TO

MENOPAUSE

Dr. Liz's

EASY GUIDE TO

MENOPAUSE

5

Simple Steps

to Balancing Your Hormones

and Feeling Like Yourself Again

Dr. Liz Lyster

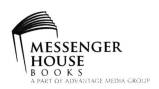

MESSENGER
HOUSE
B O O K S
A PART OF ADVANTAGE MEDIA GROUP

Published by Messenger House, Charleston, South Carolina.
Member of Advantage Media Group.

MESSENGER HOUSE is a registered trademark and the Messenger House colophon is a trademark of Advantage Media Group, Inc.

Printed in the United States of America.

ISBN: 978-1-59932-167-7
LCCN: 2009912472

This publication is designed to provide accurate and authoritative information in regard to the subject matter covered. It is sold with the understanding that the publisher is not engaged in rendering legal, accounting, or other professional services. If legal advice or other expert assistance is required, the services of a competent professional person should be sought.

Most Advantage Media Group titles are available at special quantity discounts for bulk purchases for sales promotions, premiums, fundraising, and educational use. Special versions or book excerpts can also be created to fit specific needs.

For more information, please write: Special Markets, Advantage Media Group, P.O. Box 272, Charleston, SC 29402 or call 1.866.775.1696.

Visit us online at **advantagefamily**.com

DEDICATION

This book is dedicated to my grandmother, z"l

Zelmira Silbert Vintas

ACKNOWLEDGMENTS

The experience of writing this book felt just like a pregnancy, labor, and birth. Many people helped bring it to light.

I would not have been physically able to write this book had it not been for Russ Lyster. He is a hands-on dad who balances his own work with caring for our kids, Anthony and Charlie. For this book in particular, he covered many entire afternoons and evenings while I sat at my office writing for long, uninterrupted periods of time. Thank you, Russ.

I call Sophfronia Scott my "writing coach." Her book, "Doing Business by the Book", and the webinar she taught based on this book gave me the structure, the deadlines, and the advice I needed to turn the idea for this book, which I had carried around for at least two years, into reality. She was the "doctor" who helped "deliver" this baby. The other "doctor" in attendance has been my editor Kim Hall, at Advantage Media, who always cheerfully answers my every email making yet another change. Thank you to everyone at Messenger House and Advantage Media.

My mom, Dr. Norah Gutrecht, is a pediatrician who has always been my mentor and my biggest fan. She helped me edit this book at various stages along the way. I am grateful to my mom and my dad, Dr. Jose Gutrecht, for their love and support.

I am also grateful to my patients, many of whom I surveyed and gave me invaluable input into the construction and content of this book. Thank you for sharing your stories and your lives with me. I love my job.

TABLE OF CONTENTS

INTRODUCTION

Day in and day out, I see women suffering.

Most of the time, they look really good while suffering. Who wants to look like she can't handle it all? Work, family, relationships, kids—dozens of plates spinning at the same time. She's over forty, keeping all these plates spinning, and is she taking care of herself? Maybe. Is she getting enough rest? Doubtful.

As a gynecologist specializing in menopause, hormone balance, and weight loss, my job is incredibly rewarding. Even though we see one another in the medical arena, we have a chance to talk, we develop a relationship, and we walk together through the areas of your life that matter to you. We put the physical issues that are happening in the bigger context of who you are as a woman in the best part of your life.

As an avid people-watcher, a woman over forty, a wife, and a mom of two boys, I have been through enough of my own experiences to relate to pretty much every woman I meet. Just give me a few minutes and I can find something unique and interesting about you, and about whatever experiences you are going through, or have survived.

THE CONTEXT OF BEING A WOMAN IN TODAY'S WORLD

When I take you through the evolutionary context of being a woman, you will see how nowadays we pressure ourselves excessively and unreasonably. We often feel exhausted, and inadequate that we can't make it all work all the time. For the most part, it's not our fault! (And by the way it's not men's fault either!) Once we see the design of being a woman, and identify what is happening to our bodies, we can then do an honest assessment of the situation and develop a powerful and empowering plan. I support women in doing that exploration, developing a plan, and implementing it in their lives.

Women in their forties, and certainly in their fifties and up, *are supposed* to be evaluating our lives and "growing up." We are *not supposed* to want to have a lot of sex. Women in menopause cannot (naturally) make new babies and carry on the species. Ten thousand years ago, women who got to be over forty or fifty were busy dispensing the wisdom and advice necessary to keep the culture going and the society together. At that time, if a woman of this age had sex it was because she really wanted to, maybe as part of a ritual, in which she was central, important, and incredibly appreciated. She was among the wise elders, and highly valued, not so much for her sexual attributes as for her important feminine human contribution.

MY OWN STORY

I was moseying along minding my own business when I was in my thirties. I was married, I had my two children, and I was working as an OB/GYN doctor. As I was getting ready to turn forty, my menstrual periods started changing. In my case, my periods had been coming every twenty-five days for a few years, but this was not a problem because my period was only a few days each month and it was light. A friend of mine, when I told her my cycle was that short, said "Gosh, that's like thirteen periods per year." Well, I got out my calculator and I realized that I was having *fifteen* periods per year! As my fortieth birthday approached, my periods started getting heavier. It became a real problem and something I was really not happy about. That was the beginning of my interest in what is referred to as the perimenopause (we'll come back to terminology a few times later in this book).

Here's the kicker: during the writing of this book, I decided to practice what I preach. I got a full panel of lab work done on myself, including general health tests as well as hormone tests. While I knew I was feeling warmer than everyone else in recent months, I had not had a full panel done in a couple of years. When I saw my lab results, I found out the big news: I am going into menopause! So the labor of love that is this book is by a woman who is walking the walk.

Many things led up to the writing of this book. Turning forty is a wonderful turning point in many women's lives. For me, turning forty was an eye-opening process, not just an event. It's the time when you begin to care a lot less about what others think of you and more about what you want to accomplish with your life. It's what author and coach Barbara Sher refers calls a time where you go from the life you were born into to the life you create.

It's also a time when your body starts to change at a faster pace. Our cycle changes, our metabolism changes, our hormones change. Sometimes these changes are no big deal and you can go along in your life doing your activities with little disruption. For others, the changes are more noticeable and sometimes bothersome or upsetting. As one of my best friends said, "Why is my body changing and who gave it permission to change?"

For many years as a doctor I counseled women about how to best take care of themselves. I got frustrated with this one-person-at-a-time process and enrolled at UCLA in the Executive Masters in Public Health Program for Health Professionals. My program was in the Community Health Sciences Department, in Health Education. After this program, though, I had my first son, and I have worked part-time as a doctor ever since. I only got to pursue my passion for Health Education when I had the time and energy to organize my own classes at the hospitals where I have worked. This book was born from this passion. By empowering ourselves with knowledge, we can achieve wisdom.

THE CIRCLE OF HEALTH

Many of you have gone to lectures where the speaker draws a vertical line and a horizontal line to show the different areas of life as quadrants. When I give talks, I draw two concentric circles on the board. There are still four areas: medical, nutrition, exercise, and spiritual. These four areas are not separate but rather they blend and flow into each other.

All four areas of the circle have to be explored. There is the medical area—is there a medical problem going on to explain fatigue, disrupted menstrual cycles, and so on? There is the nutritional area—what are we eating, and would my great-grandmother have recognized that snack as an actual food item?

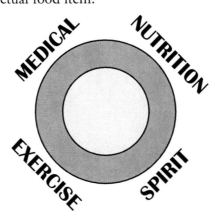

The exercise area—how much and what kind of exercise are we doing, and is it beneficial or making things worse? And last but never least, the mind/body or spiritual area—it is never the case that something is "*all* in your head" but the brain is very powerful and it *can* be the source of distress and disease. These four areas flow back and forth into each other. For example, what we eat can directly influence our moods, as can exercise. Medications can cause nutritional imbalances, resulting in new problems. These areas are not distinct—that is why I draw them around a flowing circle, and not in quadrants that give the illusion of being separate and distinct.

In this book we are going to spend most of our time in the medical area of the circle. We're going to talk about the physiological changes that are happening, how to assess these changes, and how to construct a plan of action to help your second half of your life be your best.

So, let's get started.

PART I

THE BASIC DESIGN – THE MIDLIFE WOMAN'S BODY

MENOPAUSE 101

The subtitle for this first part could be, as my friend said, "Why is my body changing and who gave it permission to change?" I also call this "a whirlwind tour through a woman's body and hormones." Before we talk about the changes happening during menopause, I want to *briefly* review the very basics of the normal menstrual cycle.

Normal menstrual cycles last between twenty-four to thirty-two days in length. We're going to take a typical menstrual cycle of twenty-eight days to make the following explanation easier to understand. Day 1 of the cycle is the first day of bleeding. During the first two weeks of the cycle, estrogen levels increase gradually, which correlates with the development of a "dominant follicle"—the one "egg of the month" that gets chosen above all the rest to develop its own follicle which grows into a cyst, a little water balloon, around that egg. During the first half of the cycle, progesterone levels stay low, and barely begin to rise just before ovulation at the mid-point of the cycle. In the middle of the twenty-eight-day cycle, a surge of stimulating hormones from the brain causes ovulation (some ovulation kits measure the LH surge). Within about twenty-four hours, the "egg of the month" gets released from the surface of the ovary, and swept into the fallopian tube where it may or may not get fertilized.

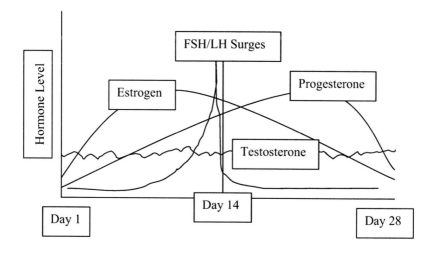

Figure 1. Hormone Levels During a 28-day Menstrual Cycle

At this point, estrogen levels start to fall, and progesterone rises, peaking mid-way through the second half of the cycle (approximately Day 21 of this cycle). This is why we measure progesterone on Day 21 of the cycle to see if ovulation has occurred properly (more on this in Step 2). If that egg does not get fertilized, progesterone levels fall, which destabilizes the lining of the uterus (endometrium) and triggers the start of the menstrual bleeding. If the egg does get fertilized, the ovary continues to produce progesterone (get it?—pro-gesterone = pro-gestation) until the placenta grows and takes over hormone production.

Now let's talk about testosterone, which is produced in small amounts by the adrenal glands and the ovaries. In the "pre-menstrual" days (think premenstrual syndrome or PMS now)—the days before the period starts—the female hormones estrogen and progesterone are falling or have fallen, and the stable level of testosterone is now relatively higher (see Figure 1). Some women experience levels of testosterone as being out of balance with the female hormones, and they feel the irritability and aggressiveness often reported as part of PMS.

Now, there is a concept going on here called *feedback* that is important to keep in mind for this and other hormone discussions we will be having. Our brains and our bodies are always in an amazing state of feedback—stimulating hormones are released by the brain, and the organs they affect make their hormones, which feed back on the brain and cause the stimulating hormones to subside (see Figure 2). This diagram illustrates three of the many feedback loops. The brain releases FSH—follicle-stimulating hormone. FSH stimulates the ovaries to make estrogen. The estrogen feeds back in a "loop" to the brain, causing the release of FSH to go back down. The same area of the brain releases TSH—thyroid stimulating hormone—which causes the thyroid gland to produce its hormones, which feed back to the brain. The third loop shown here is the brain releasing ACTH – adrenocorticotropic hormone—which stimulates the adrenal glands to produce their hormones, which also feed back in the way we have discussed. How the precise levels are controlled is a miracle of hormone receptors and the body's biochemistry, or what I often call "the body's wisdom."

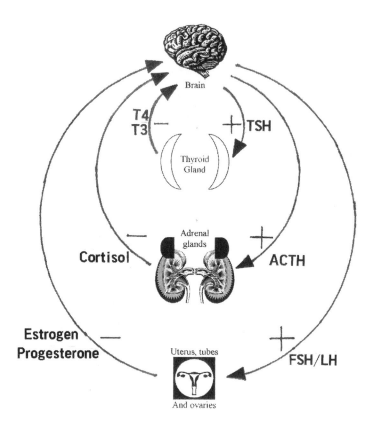

Figure 2. Basic Hormone Feedback Loops in Women

Now, only for the purposes of this explanation, I want to tell you about one more hormone, and then you can forget you ever knew about this hormone. It is called *inhibin*. Pre-menopausal ovaries go along in life making a constant level of inhibin, which feeds back on the brain, and controls the FSH level, which in turn controls the ovulation/menstruation cycle.

When the perimenopause phase of a woman's life begins, ovarian function starts to become what I call "less reliable." The quality of the progesterone production associated with ovulation is lower, and women often start to feel more mood changes during the cycle. When things continue to progress towards menopause, ovulation may not happen on schedule and the period becomes irregular. If ovulation does not happen, she may skip periods entirely and, like Stockard Channing says in the movie Grease, feel like "a broken typewriter."

When the ovarian function is really declining (the next phase after "less reliable"), the amount of inhibin drops further, and the Follicle Stimulating Hormone (FSH) level starts to go up and stay up. The FSH level is one of the main markers for menopause on blood work. (However, as we will discuss in Steps 2 and 3, you cannot declare that a woman is perimenopausal or in menopause only by this test.) Why does the FSH go up? First, it rises because inhibin falls. There is less inhibin in the feedback loop, so more FSH gets produced by the brain. Think of the higher FSH like a taskmaster—the FSH says, "Come on, ovaries! You can do this! You've got to try harder!" At first, more FSH does, in fact, cause the ovaries to make more estrogen, which leads to an excess of estrogen, causing its own fun set of symptoms like breast tenderness and fluid retention. (We'll talk more about this in Step 1, when we discuss these and many other menopause symptoms.)

In time, the ovaries stop ovulating completely and, at that point, no longer make progesterone. Then they eventually stop making estrogen. The last to go is testosterone. At this point, she may experience a relative excess of testosterone, which can cause facial hair growth, acne, and irritability. Eventually, this too will diminish, and all symptoms settle down—she is (at last) fully in menopause. This whole process usually takes between two and eight years.

It's not hard to see how surgical menopause, the entering of a woman into menopause by removal of both of her ovaries, can be abrupt and, therefore, even more difficult for her than if she had several years to adjust to the stages of progression of menopause.

LET'S AGREE ON SOME TERMINOLOGY

At this point, we have already bandied about a few terms about menopause, and I want to get us all on the same page. Many people use these terms in different ways, and I find the following definitions most useful:

Pre-menopause: During what I call the pre-menopause years, a woman is having her period on a pretty regular monthly basis, with some normal variation due to stress, pregnancy, and post-partum. She feels well overall hormonally, with normal variations during the month related to the hormone fluctuations during the cycle.

Perimenopause: I find it helpful to women to use this term very broadly. Starting as early as around age thirty-five (more typically after age forty), a woman may begin to experience changes and symptoms in her body that are hormonally caused. We will discuss these symptoms in detail in Step 1, but overall, she is having periods, even though they may be irregular. In other words, if *anything* is happening beyond regular periods and overall feeling hormonally stable, I call it peri-menopause. Medical textbooks say the perimenopause can last from two to eight years, but as you can tell from my broad definition, it can last even longer for some women.

Menopausal transition: I apply this term to either of the following: (1) the periods are very irregular and getting farther apart (skipping one or more months at a time), or (2) symptoms are becoming disruptive (such as hot flashes that disrupt her day, or night sweats that disrupt her sleep). There are a few lucky women who go through the menopausal transition very smoothly, who enjoy their "private summers," are able to compensate for any lack of sleep, and just generally do okay. (If you are one of these lucky women, you must not brag to your friends. That's like women who brag about how quick, easy, and painless their vaginal deliveries were.)

Menopause: The technical definition of menopause is *one whole year with no periods.* I wish I had a dollar for every woman I've seen in my office who got a period after a gap of eleven months and twenty-nine days. I consider a woman to be fully in menopause when she has not had periods for at least one year, and she is no longer having severe symptoms related to menopause (this is as judged by *her*).

The average age of menopause in the United States is fifty-one years of age, but this can have a really wide range. Also, this only refers to the average age of the period stopping completely. Symptoms related to menopause can start years before and can take quite a few more years to settle down in many women.

Now that we're on the same page with this terminology, let's talk about what I call "The Big Four" of women's hormones.

WOMEN'S HORMONES—THE BIG FOUR

Now we're going to focus on four hormones that are not, in fact, the most important hormones in the human body. They are, however, the four hormones that enable us to look and feel feminine or masculine, as the case may be. After we discuss The Big Four, I'll further address cortisol and insulin, the two hormones essential for survival whose variations in level dramatically affect our metabolism, how we feel, and how we function. The four hormones that I call The Big Four are (drum roll, please): estrogen, progesterone, testosterone, and DHEA. Let's talk about them one at a time.

ESTROGEN
— the lead actor (actress?) on the female hormone stage

This hormone is the major hormone in women responsible for female characteristics: breast development, follicle and egg development in the ovaries, light hair growth (as compared to men), and fat distribution around the breasts and hips leading to the female body contour.

Estrogen has effects on almost every tissue in the body, from the brain and skin, to blood vessels, bone, and the genital organs. Estrogen particularly affects hormonally responsive tissues such as the lining of the vagina, the lining of the uterus, and the base of the bladder. Estrogen affects the brain with regard to mental clarity and the temperature regulation center in the brainstem.

Estrogen also affects the water balance in the body by causing fluid retention in the cells. The right amount of estrogen causes the

PART I

right balance of softness and firmness in the tissues throughout the body. This is how estrogen affects the appearance of skin. In high amounts, such as during pregnancy, estrogen also causes darker pigmentation of the skin.

Estrogen preserves bone density, slows down the motility of the bowel, increases blood clotting, and causes favorable changes in lipids, such as increasing high-density lipoproteins (HDL or "good" cholesterol) and lowering low-density lipoproteins (LDL or "bad" cholesterol).

Estrogen is produced and released in the body in several ways. It is secreted by the ovaries, mainly during the first half of the menstrual cycle, also called the "follicular phase." By conversion, estrogen can also be made in other metabolic pathways from other hormones. It is secreted by fat tissue in this way (by conversion from another hormone). We will come back to this point after we discuss the three other hormones in this section.

Estrogen occurs in the body in three forms, according to the number of a certain side chain on the estrogen molecule: estrone has ONE of these side chains, estradiol has TWO of the side chains, and estriol has THREE. Estradiol is secreted by the ovaries into the bloodstream, converted into estrone in the liver, which goes back into the blood and is made into estriol, which is then changed into a form excreted by the kidneys into the urine. Overall, these three forms occur in balance in a woman's body.

Estradiol is the most potent of these forms. Estrone is the weakest. The amounts of each type change during a woman's life. Estrone is the most common form in menopause. Estradiol is the most active overall, controlling the first half of the menstrual cycle, and is the most common form made for pharmaceutical use. Estriol is made in large amounts during pregnancy.

As we discussed earlier, estrogen feeds back in a loop to the brain. When the estrogen level is higher, the amount of Follicle Stimulating Hormone will go down. This finely tuned system usually ensures that only one egg will be released during a typical menstrual cycle.

Estrogen stimulates the development of the lining of the uterus during the first half of the menstrual cycle. If no pregnancy occurs, normal events lead to the regularly scheduled shedding of the lining in the form of menstrual bleeding. If ovulation does not happen, as is common in the perimenopausal time and later, estrogen can continue to exert its influence, resulting in continued growth of the uterine lining. Eventually, bleeding will occur, and it may be heavy or prolonged. Doctors call this "unopposed estrogen," and, in some cases, this can cause precancerous and cancerous changes in the lining of the uterus. In most cases, this is easy to prevent by "opposing," or balancing, the estrogen with some form of progesterone. We can now turn to discussing estrogen's balancing hormone, progesterone.

PROGESTERONE
— the "sleepy, feel-contented" hormone

Now let's talk about the other hormone, which along with estrogen, is responsible for feeling and cycling in a normal female way. As the name implies, the main function of progesterone is to support the lining of the uterus in the second half of the menstrual cycle in preparation for pregnancy (gestation). If the egg released during ovulation gets fertilized, the ovary will continue to make progesterone until the placenta gets big enough to take over.

Progesterone influences breast development and the uterine lining during the second half of the menstrual cycle by stabilizing the stimulating effects of estrogen. It acts as a natural diuretic, by influencing the kidneys to release water (the opposite of retaining water). Progesterone affects carbohydrate metabolism by controlling insulin response. It slightly increases body temperature, probably through the temperature-regulation center of the brain. It affects the sensitivity of lung ventilation, contributing to the shortness of breath many women feel during pregnancy. Last but not least, progesterone in its naturally occurring form causes a sedating effect on the brain. For most women, it is high levels of progesterone that gives pregnant women a feeling of calm, contented sleepiness.

In a normal menstrual cycle, progesterone is the dominant hormone during the second half of the cycle, after ovulation has occurred. If the egg released during that ovulation does not get fertilized, the progesterone level will fall. This withdrawal of the progesterone then results in menstrual bleeding. When progesterone production is not normal, the results can include difficulty conceiving, menstrual irregularities, mood changes, or disrupted sleep.

In hormone replacement therapy, progesterone balances the stimulating effect of estrogen. When a woman has had a hysterectomy and does not have her uterus, we are taught in mainstream medical training that when she needs estrogen to help with menopausal symptoms, she does not need any progesterone. We are now learning that for many women this is not correct. If no progesterone is provided, she may have symptoms of estrogen excess, which we will discuss in Step 1.

It is important to note that most pharmaceutically made forms of progesterone are properly called *progestins*. A progestin has a side chain on the progesterone molecule that changes its effects. For the purposes of our discussion, when I use the word "progesterone" I am referring to a form that is identical to what is made by the ovaries. While progesterone in its natural form has many benefits, progestins, especially in menopause, are associated with several important problematic side effects. We will go over this in detail in Step 4, when we discuss hormone therapy options.

TESTOSTERONE
— the "confidence hormone"

You know how most men seem to saunter through life, overall feeling pretty darn good about themselves? This is a function of testosterone. Many of my patients tell me they never knew women even have testosterone in their bodies. For women, the right level of testosterone gives a feeling of self-confidence.

Testosterone is one of a group of androgens, which cause normal hair growth at puberty, and also affect metabolism. In women, testosterone is released by the ovaries and the adrenal glandsin overall small amounts. In the adrenal glands, it is a metabolic product resulting from DHEA (which we will talk about next). In the right amount, testosterone enhances women's libido, ability to reach orgasm, energy level, muscle tone, mental clarity, and overall sense of well-being.

In the perimenopausal time, if other hormone levels are low, there may be relatively higher amounts of testosterone. For example, when the menopausal transition is mostly (but not completely) finished, there may be relatively low amounts of estrogen and progesterone, but the ovaries may still be making a little bit of testosterone. This is when women experience masculine effects such as acne or facial hair growth. A relative excess of testosterone can also cause mood disturbances. We saw all of this in earlier (in Figure 1), showing the same relative hormone changes during a regular menstrual cycle. In great excess, testosterone can give women virilizing side effects such as a deepening of the voice. We will talk about this in greater detail in our discussions of symptoms (Step 1) and hormone therapy (Step 4).

DHEA
— the major player in women's sex drive

DHEA is short for (get ready for it) dehydroepiandrosterone. Luckily, you never need to remember that again. DHEA is made by the adrenal glands. The amount of DHEA made reaches a peak level at about age twenty-five to thirty and gradually declines after that. DHEA metabolizes into estrogen and testosterone and is the major source of testosterone in women. DHEA results in an increased feeling of energy, well-being, and libido. As with excess testosterone, too much production or supplementation of DHEA can result in masculinizing side effects including excess facial hair growth, acne, and irritability.

DHEA is produced by the adrenals in inverse proportion to cortisol. For example, if the adrenals release cortisol in response to stress, thencortisol secretion is high, and production of DHEA will usually be low. Anything that can raise the cortisol level can decrease the DHEA level (see below in the discussion of cortisol).

DHEA is easy to measure on a blood test, which will be discussed in detail in Step 2. This hormone is also easy to replace with an oral supplement (over-the-counter) or in a compounded product (by prescription). We will also go into detail about this in Step 4 when we discuss treatment options.

MAJOR HORMONES

As I said earlier, the four hormones we have discussed are not the most important hormones in the body. Let me talk briefly about three substances that are critically important to both men and women.

The first major hormone that I will mention briefly here is *cortisol.* We mentioned in our discussion of DHEA that cortisol is made by the adrenal glands. Cortisol (and its related hormone cortisone) is critically important for regulating the metabolism of fats, carbohydrates, and proteins, as well as sodium and potassium. Fluid balance (water retention in and around the cells) is controlled mainly through sodium movement in and out of the cells of the body, and cortisol affects this cellular movement of water.

Many things affect cortisol production including stress, foods we eat, and medical illnesses. Foods that increase cortisol levels include all of the "white" foods, including white sugar, white bread, and white rice.

The second major hormone to mention briefly here is *insulin*. This hormone has almost one entire page just in my medical dictionary (and has entire books and careers devoted to it). This hormone is produced by the pancreas and is essential for the metabolism of glucose and maintaining proper blood sugar levels. Too much or too little insulin is life-threatening. Insulin affects glucose storage in liver and muscle tissue and prevents breakdown of proteins. For our purposes, it can be seen as causing our bodies to retain calories, which are stored for later use.

Finally (for now), a brief word about *cholesterol*. Why am I mentioning cholesterol? Because you can't live without it! Cholesterol is the basic building block for *all* of the "Big Four" hormones, and for several others we won't spend time on here (you can go to http://www.drlizmd.com/DrLizBlog1/dr-lizs-easy-guide-to-menopause/metabolismchart - for more detailed information on the miracle that is hormone metabolism). What's important here is to realize that it is *not* healthy to have too low of a cholesterol level. We'll get more specific about this is Step 2.

So, if you're ready to dive in to a discussion of the symptoms of perimenopause and menopause then turn the page and let's take Step 1.

PART II

THE 5 SIMPLE STEPS

STEP 1

IDENTIFY YOUR SYMPTOMS - EASY GUIDE TO MENOPAUSE SYMPTOMS

The onset of perimenopause and menopause can be heralded by a wide variety of symptoms. Sorting through what is and what is not normal for this time in your life is our first step and our first priority. One of my patients, Anne, was a walking catalog of symptoms during the menopausal transition, which was apparent when she wrote:

"Between 2003 and 2006, I had the following things develop: weight gain (I had weighed just about the same since I was a teenager, except when I was pregnant with my son), difficulty sleeping through the night, profuse sweating at night for the few days before the start of my period, and adult acne on my face and back. Then between 2006 and 2009, I had significant weight gain, continued difficulty sleeping through the night, continued sweating during the night, but now also profuse sweating during the day (sometimes I thought I was going to pass out), feeling tired and a lack of energy, little to no interest in sex, and aching knees and joints throughout my body. My last actual period was in the summer of 2008."

Needless to say, each woman is different, so this guide is organized from "head to toe." Take note that this guide is not presenting these symptoms in order of importance or in order of commonness. Therefore, you will need to cross-reference this guide with the "summary by age-decade" list below. Also, keep in mind that women are beautiful complex beings, and areas of our bodies are often not clearly defined and separate from other areas. It's all inter-connected.

I am always saying to my patients and my audiences: **LIFE IS ABOUT QUALITY OF LIFE.** So, I want you to use this information to assess and prioritize what is most affecting your quality of life, and go from there. When women do this regularly, they will feel empowered and uplifted. When doctors do this regularly, they will receive a lot of thank-yous, and I won't have to hear so often, "You're the first doctor who has ever really listened to me!"

Summary by age-decade:

AGE DECADE	MAIN HORMONAL CHANGE	MAIN SYMPTOMS
40 to 50	Perimenopause usually starts	Menstrual cycle changes Mood Changes Sleep disturbances Abdominal weight gain
50 to 60	Menstrual periods stop	Menstruation stops Hot flashes, night sweats Sleep disrupted Abdominal weight gain
60 +	Intensity of hormonal symptoms drops	Vaginal dryness Abdominal weight gain

40 TO 50

The "perimenopause" is technically considered to be two to eight years before the actual stopping of the menstrual period, so it most commonly begins within this age-decade. The changes I list here can start even earlier, and do not correlate with the actual age at which menopause will occur (menstrual periods completely gone for one whole year). In other words, if you start having symptoms at age thirty-eight, it doesn't mean you will stop having periods by eight years after that. Also, family history is not a good predictor of when a woman will go into menopause.

Most common changes during this decade: menstrual cycle changes, mood changes, sleep disturbance and abdominal weight gain.

50 TO 60

It is during this decade that most women in the United States stop having their menstrual period. The average age is fifty-one years. It is also during this decade that temperature symptoms and sleep disruption will usually be at their most bothersome.

Most common changes: menstrual period stops, hot flashes/night sweats, disrupted sleep, abdominal weight gain.

60 AND UP

By age sixty, most women experience a significant drop in the intensity of menopausal symptoms. Many women during this decade will experience a complete resolution of menopause-related symptoms.

Most common (remaining) symptoms related to menopause: vaginal dryness, abdominal weight gain.

So, let's start at the top.

THE HEAD

It was hard for me to limit what to include in this section, because the brain is so incredibly important. The phrase "it's all in your head" is awful for several reasons. First, the obvious, it's patronizing and insulting. But more importantly, it ignores the *power of the mind.* People experience a sensory phenomenon known as phantom pains in amputated limbs. Does this mean they are crazy? Of course not! What it means is that the pathways in the brain that lead to an interpretation and an experience of pain in that area are being triggered, even though there is no longer the original stimulus coming from where the hand used to be. As this illustrates, the mind is a powerful thing.

The following are questions I am often asked by my patients, going from head to toe.

Q. Why is my hair leaving my scalp and eyebrows and landing on my upper lip and chin?

A. Hair excess or hair loss: At midlife, as we have discussed, there begin to be relative changes in the levels of hormones. There can be a higher ratio of androgens to estrogens. In some women, this can result in a relative excess of free testosterone, which increases the growth of facial hair. For other women, the excess of testosterone can result in a type of male pattern baldness of the scalp. Also, in many women, androgens affect the scalp by shortening the growth phase of the hair follicle growth cycle, which causes the hair to have a finer, thinner texture. There are significant differences between individuals and between racial or ethnic groups in amounts of facial and body hair.

Other causes of hair loss include medical problems such as thyroid dysfunction and nutritional problems such as a diet that is too high in refined sugars. A poor diet and excess body fat not only cause general health problems, but can also contribute to hair excess or hair loss by shifting the hormonal balance towards androgen production.

Q. Why am I now getting terrible headaches?

A. Headaches: As we have discussed, beginning in perimenopause, hormones levels change relative to each other. A relative excess of estrogen can cause headaches. As I mentioned earlier, it has been traditional in gynecology to treat women who have had a hysterectomy with only estrogen for menopause-related symptoms. In this scenario, women may experience headaches, breast tenderness, and joint pain due to the fluid retention caused by estrogen not balanced by progesterone. The other symptoms mentioned here are further discussed below.

There are also many women who get headaches and even migraines when there is a relative lack of estrogen. For example, women who get migraines on their period (menstrual migraines) often benefit from a small amount of estrogen during their menstrual period. There are several low-dose birth control pills that contain low amounts of estrogen during the menstrual week (which is usually a week of placebo pills containing no hormones at all).

In summary, too much or too little estrogen can cause headaches in women. Because the levels of estrogen may be going up and down dramatically during the perimenopause and menopause, headaches are a common symptom.

Q. Why am I forgetful? Am I going crazy or losing my memory?

A. Mental fogginess/memory loss: This is not your imagination! Scientific studies are now documenting that this is a real phenomenon related to menopause. One recent study showed that women approaching menopause (late forties and early fifties in age) had lower performance on memory testing. The good news is that their performance improved to baseline levels after their menopausal transition was completed (by about mid-fifties in age). The cause is not precisely clear, but it might be a function of lower estrogen levels, and possibly also lower testosterone levels. It can also be due to being tired from disrupted sleep.

Q. Why am I suddenly so cranky for no reason?

A. Mood changes: This is one of the most common complaints I hear from women in their forties. This is usually the perimenopausal time for them, and here's what is happening. Even if you are having regular monthly menstrual periods, what I call the quality of progesterone production during the second half of the cycle is decreasing during these years. Most scientific studies of pre-menopausal progesterone levels have focused on women who are trying to get pregnant and/or retain pregnancies (i.e. not miscarry). In these studies, women were given progesterone gel to use vaginally to use during the second half of the cycle (after ovulation and hopefully after fertilization had occurred), and during the first few weeks of the pregnancy. Many studies have not shown an improvement over using a placebo gel. The mainstream medical community behaves in an interesting way on this subject. Even though these studies would normally lead doctors not to use the progesterone gel, they continue to do so. This is smart, in my opinion, because it is likely that we just don't yet know how to properly measure progesterone levels and progesterone receptor activity, so we don't know how to predict exactly which women will benefit from this treatment.

Most women report an increased feeling of peace and calmness during pregnancy. This is a function of progesterone. So, on the subject of the mood disturbances that happen to women in their perimenopausal years, if the quality of progesterone production is less, especially during the second half of the cycle, mood will suffer. Women will often benefit from low doses of progesterone supplementation at this point in their lives (we'll talk about this further in Step 4). Also, if mood changes are due to lack of sleep, improvement in sleep quality and quantity will improve mood.

Q. Help! I can't sleep!

A. Disrupted sleep: Let's recall for a moment the contextual issue we discussed at the beginning of this book. The average forty-plus-year-old woman ten thousand years ago was not raising her own small children or adolescents. Most women nowadays are busy with activities and stresses that impair sleep hygiene. Hot flashes and night sweats may wake a woman up from sleep. Less noticeably, they can disrupt sleep cycles/REM sleep in a way that doesn't wake her up enough to realize she's awake, but disturbs her sleep quality enough to have her feel tired during the day. I have heard this from women who say they get enough hours of sleep but still feel exhausted. I have had patients tell me they thought they were getting enough sleep, but had a sleep study done and were told they were actually waking several times during the night. The sleep study technology detects temperature changes during the night that interfere with restorative sleep patterns.

There is also what I call "ambient stress." Emails, phone calls, and all sorts of other forms of communication are going on around us constantly. There is also constant noise around us, including some we are not even consciously aware of, such as from airplanes and power lines. Our lives span several time zones, with family and work obligations spread out   across the country and around the world. I have a patient who gets home from her workday, and then begins taking care of calls from the Hong Kong office of her company, because it's the morning there!

More and more people are now appreciating the importance of good sleep habits and good sleep quality. For example, adequate sleep is essential for long-term weight control (we'll come back to this topic).

Q. Why am I waking up soaked?

A. Hot flashes/night sweats: The temperature regulation center of the brain is in the brainstem (at the base of the skull at the top of the spinal cord). This is where hot flashes and night sweats originate. It is not a direct function of dropping estrogen levels, as many believe. In fact, there may be increased levels of estrogen in the body when women begin to experience hot flashes. It seems to be a question of irregularity in levels of estrogen that affects this brainstem center and causes temperature fluctuation.

During perimenopause, night sweats may respond well to progesterone supplementation. During menopausal transition and menopause, if women are having hot flashes during the day, and/or night sweats, these symptoms usually respond best to estrogen supplementation. We will go into more detail on this in Step 4.

Q. Why am I always exhausted?

A. Fatigue: Here we have another symptom of perimenopause and menopause that defies pigeon-holing into one part of the body. There are two categories of tired. The first is physical—not enough sleep, disrupted sleep, and medical disorders that cause fatigue. When you feel this kind of tiredness, it is not usually accompanied by thoughts and feelings of exhaustion. The second is mental—it's physical tiredness plus gloomy thoughts or feelings. It's the difference between how it feels staying up to get your taxes done versus staying up to plan a vacation. Or, the difference between feeling that things are not going to work out as opposed to the feeling that things are great and life is wonderful—when you feel great about life, you just generally feel a lot less tired!

If a woman is woken by night sweats or children, she may feel the first type of tired. If she is dealing with mental stressors during this phase of her life, she may have more of the second type of fatigue. Many of my patients have both. Also, tiredness leading to lack of exercise sets up a downward spiral to feeling even more tired.

Then of course there are medical causes of fatigue, including thyroid disease, anemia, cancer, andadrenal disease. The condition of adrenal fatigue will be addressed in a moment.

THE BREASTS

Q. "My breasts are killing me!"

A. Breast tenderness: This is typically due to a relative excess of estrogen. That is to say, too much estrogen or too little progesterone. As we have discussed, this could be from more estrogen being released from the ovaries in perimenopause (remember that FSH—follicle-stimulating hormone—trying harder to get those ovaries to work) or from decreased progesterone production, especially during the second half of the cycle.

Also, we mentioned that most doctors will prescribe only estrogen replacement for women who have had a hysterectomy. Some of these women will have symptoms of estrogen excess, and most progestins prescribed by doctors will not relieve these symptoms (but progesterone will). More on this in Step 4.

THE BELLY

Q. I'm doing everything the same, so why am I gaining weight around my middle?

A. Abdominal weight gain: We're now around the middle of the body. The two adrenal glands are very small and extremely important glands. Each gland is about the size of the top part of your thumb, and sits atop each kidney. We cannot live without adrenal glands.

Mainstream medicine is mostly only aware of extreme disorders of the adrenals—too much (Cushing's disease) or too little (Addison's disease) adrenal hormone production. The fact is that the adrenal glands can be dysfunctional at what we call a "sub-clinical" level—the usual lab tests that doctors are familiar with to evaluate the adrenals will be within a normal reference range, but the person will still have symptoms of adrenal deficiency.

Adrenal fatigue is the condition in which stress or diet causes relatively excessive amounts of cortisol to be released by the adrenal glands, and DHEA levels are decreased. It is the excess cortisol that gives us that belly pooch. This is not simply a function of weight gain on the outside of the body (just under the skin where we can pinch it). There is water retention in the tissues and fat deposition around the internal organs as well. That is why abdominal obesity is also called visceral adiposity, and is very dangerous to our health.

THE PELVIS

Q. Why is my sex drive so low?

A. Low libido: Where should this symptom go? I could have put it up near brain because the two biggest sex organs are the skin and the brain. We'll talk about dry skin below, under vaginal dryness. So here we are again, with several levels of causes for decreased sex drive (libido). We have erratic (perimenopausal) or declining (menopausal transition and menopause) hormone levels, disrupted sleep, and physical discomfort in our erogenous zones (breasts, vagina). We have contextual challenges—evaluating life purpose, and maybe a sex partner who is doing their own life-evaluating (if there is a sex partner in the picture at this point).

As we discussed before, in an evolutionary context, a woman at fifty or more years of age is not supposed to want to have that much sex! She cannot (without technology) make new babies and carry on the species. Her fifty-year-old male counterpart on the other hand, is still able to make babies quite effectively and so it is biologically appropriate for his sex drive to stay higher (although usually lower than his previous level). If he has any inclination to have sex with younger "reproductive age" women, this makes evolutionary sense, whether or not it is good in society.

In women, DHEA is the most important hormone for promotion of sexual interest, sexual response, and sexual function (ability to achieve orgasm). Levels of production in the ovaries and adrenal glands of DHEA (which metabolizes into testosterone) normally fall gradually over a woman's lifespan. This decline starts by around age thirty. By the time a woman reaches perimenopause or menopause, levels of DHEA may be very low. Also, low DHEA and testosterone levels may be present in adrenal fatigue, which in turn can be caused by poor diet and/or stress. The levels of DHEA and testosterone are easily measured on a blood test (see Step 2).

But let me add a big "however"! As I said, the two biggest sex organs are the skin and the brain. In the case of women over forty, I think the brain may be the biggest issue. How much is on our minds at this point? How are our marriages/relationships? Are we raising small children? Teenagers? Are we sleeping enough? Is it good-quality sleep? These are important factors that directly affect hormonal balance.

Q. Why are my nice, regular periods going haywire?

A. Changes in the menstrual cycle: This is, in my medical opinion, a clear marker of the perimenopausal stage of life. The ovarian hormone inhibin declines gradually over a woman's lifetime (usually starting in her thirties, although this varies from woman to woman—also see our discussion in Part I). When inhibin decreases, FSH increases. Initially, this causes the ovaries to try harder, and release more estrogen. The changes in follicle growth and ovulation cause the changes in the menstrual cycle. Also, as we said before, the quality of progesterone production is less reliable at this time of life which also deregulates the cycle. (See Part I to review the details.)

There are now several good studies that show that if the period is changing in quality (heavier or lighter, longer or shorter) but still coming on, more or less, a monthly schedule, then this is par for the course and probably not indicative of any underlying problem. If the menstrual periods are getting further apart, and not getting heavier, then this is also normal for perimenopause.

However, if the periods are getting heavier and also irregular or more than once a month, then further evaluation of the endometrium (lining of the uterus) might be necessary. Only about five percent of endometrial cancers occur in women under age fifty. While it is not common, it is easy to rule it out with an office biopsy of the endometrium. Sometimes, your gynecologist will want to do a more involved assessment of your endometrium, including a special ultrasound or direct visualization (hysteroscopy). Many gynecologists will want to do an endometrial biopsy in women over forty having menstrual problems; some doctors have a lower threshold and want a biopsy in women over thirty-five having these problems. (You can find more information about these procedures on my Web site at http://www.drlizmd.com/DrLizBlog1/dr-lizs-easy-guide-to-menopause/evaluation.)

Q. Why does my vagina feel like paper?

A. Vaginal dryness: This is mainly a function of lack of estrogen reaching the vaginal tissues. Remember I mentioned that some women can have excess estrogen production during the perimenopause? I have seen some women with estrogen excess symptoms (including women already on hormone therapy) who still have vaginal dryness. This is a lack of estrogen reaching the cells of the vaginal skin. This can happen especially if vaginal dryness developed before a woman started replacing estrogen; her thinned vaginal lining lost the tiny blood vessels needed for estrogen to reach those cells.

The cells of the lower part of the urethra and base of the bladder also respond to estrogen. Women with severe dryness of these tissues can have increased bladder complaints, such as more frequent urinary tract infections. Urine leakage is not usually directly due to lack of estrogen to the bladder base, but it can be made worse by lack of estrogen to these tissues.

It is not just the surface of the skin in these areas that is affected. It's the thickness and the elasticity of the underlying tissue of the vaginal walls (and base of the bladder) that is decreased with a lack of estrogen. If vaginal discomfort results in avoiding having sex, then a downward spiral can happen. Less use of your vagina can result in further loss of elasticity and de-conditioning of the tissues. It can really become a "use it or lose it" situation.

OTHER

Q. Are my achy joints and dry eyes due to menopause?

A. These symptoms are common during menopause but may or may not be directly hormonally caused.

Joint pains: There are many possible causes for generalized discomfort in joints such as shoulders, hips, and knees. Medical problems can include autoimmune diseases, injuries, and arthritis. Obesity can not only put physical strain on the body, but we now know that excess adipose tissue causes hormonal fluctuations that cause inflammation and harm the body tissues. For our purposes however, I will note that perimenopausal and menopausal women who have a new onset of generalized joint pain with no other identifiable cause may have estrogen excess causing fluid retention in the body. I have had many patients with diffuse joint pain respond well to hormone balancing with progesterone (see Step 4).

Visual changes/dry eyes: Eye related symptoms are also generally not caused by hormonal changes. For example, changes in visual acuity are often a normal part of the aging process. Dry eyes can be caused by autoimmune disorders. However, I have had several patients with these symptoms, especially dry eyes, who have an improvement when their hormones are replaced in an appropriate and balanced manner. This is probably related to correcting the fluid balance in the cells of her body.

WHAT'S NOT NORMAL FOR MENOPAUSE?

Let's turn for a moment to some symptoms and body changes that often occur in women in midlife that are not directly caused by going through menopause. In other words, the following items should not be considered a normal part of menopause. Normal symptoms of menopause may clear up on their own with time and no treatment. The following items should not be expected to resolve on their own and deserve special evaluation and attention.

Depression: Feelings of sadness and stress are common among women in the perimenopausal and menopausal age ranges. However, the clinical diagnosis of depression is not a normal part of the menopausal transition. Defined briefly, depression includes a variety of disturbances that happen for a least a two-week period. These disturbances include both mental and physical signs and symptoms. The mental symptoms include feeling depressed or sad and tearful. The physical changes can include agitation, decreased appetite, fast heartbeat, and fatigue. These signs and symptoms impair the person's ability to function normally in their life.

Depression is more commonly reported in women than in men. Depression has many causes including a chemical imbalance in the brain and a family history indicating possible genetic factors. It can be triggered by other medical conditions or by medications and it can also be caused or made worse by the use of drugs and alcohol.

My first concern when a patient says she is feeling depressed is to find out about her sleep quality. A woman who is exhausted has very limited capacity to handle stress, even normal daily life stress. The diagnosis can also be made difficult because women in the perimenopausal and menopausal age ranges can be going through quite a few life changes at the same time that can cause excess stress.

I see many women in their forties and up who were seen by a doctor, and offered an antidepressant before being offered hormonal evaluation and treatment. By the same token, it is very important to diagnose and treat depression if it persists after menopausal symptoms have been evaluated, treated, and resolved.

Palpitations: Just as with depression, women have reported to me feeling a fast heartbeat, often accompanied by anxiety. It can be hard to tell whether the anxiety is causing the palpitations or whether feeling a fast heartbeat causes her to feel scared and anxious about her health. It is important in this situation to see a general doctor (internist or family practitioner) for a thorough cardiac evaluation.

Abnormal thyroid function: Thyroid dysfunction is also more common in women, occurring up to eight times as often in women as in men. In medical school, doctors learn to rely on one blood test in order to evaluate thyroid function. This test is called TSH—thyroid stimulating hormone. This hormone is released by the brain and goes to the thyroid gland, which then makes thyroid hormone in two forms which are referred to as T-3 and T-4. To do a full evaluation of the thyroid requires checking levels of at least these three hormones. This is discussed in further detail in Step 2.

Low functioning thyroid (also referred to as "sluggish thyroid") can cause a woman to feel tired, have irregular menstrual periods, and have other related changes in hair and skin. Therefore, these symptoms can be confused with some of the normal symptoms that occur during menopause. Because of this, we have to be sure to evaluate thyroid function as part of a full hormone workup.

Thinning bones: Another condition that affects women in the perimenopausal and menopausal age ranges is osteopenia or osteoporosis. A decrease in bone density must also be evaluated and treated as its own entity, and not accepted simply as a normal part of aging. Osteoporosis experts and advocates promote the prevention of hip and vertebral fractures as a top priority for a long and healthy life.

Women are at a disadvantage with bone density because due to our smaller frames we do not build as high of a peak bone density as men usually do. Peak bone density is reached by the age of late teens or early twenties. Lifetime calcium intake also affects bone density. The optimal uptake of calcium into the bones happens when there are normal levels of estrogen circulating through the blood. This means that in menopause whether or not a woman is still producing or replacing estrogen affects the dose of calcium that she needs to take to maintain healthy bone structure. A good level of vitamin D is also essential to maintaining bone density. If there is not enough vitamin D, then even if there is good bone structure, calcium will not be deposited correctly into that structure, which can also result in bone fractures.

Now that we have been through a whirlwind tour touching on the most common symptoms women experience during perimenopause and menopause, you can assess your symptoms, put them in order of priority, and be able to work with your doctor to develop a plan of action.

Next, we take Step 2, in which we take adetailed look at the laboratory evaluation of hormone levels. You'll need some of this information to develop your personal plan of action. So let's move on and learn information about lab tests that assess perimenopause and menopause.

STEP 2

GET THOROUGH LAB TESTING

TESTS FOR MENOPAUSE

There are almost as many ways to measure hormones levels as there are ways to skin a cat. Not surprisingly, people disagree on the best way to measure hormone levels.

Several factors affect the choice of how to measures hormone levels. First, it depends on the hormone being measured. If the hormone has a very short half-life, that is to say it lasts for a very short time in the body once it is made, then it is very hard to measure. The same applies if the hormone has a very short distance to travel in the body; it affects cells very near where it is made. As an analogy, if you are a pizza delivery person, but you only deliver pizza to your next-door neighbor, or maybe even only to yourself, then it's harder to catch you during delivery to count the pizzas.

Second, most hormones undergo daily, monthly, or longer variations in their levels. For example, when measuring a hormone released with a circadian rhythm, a regular repeating pattern every twenty-four hours, the time of day will affect the results. Measuring adrenal hormone levels is the classic example of this—normal cortisol levels vary in predictable ranges during the day. If the hormone variation is over the course of the month, such as in the cases of estrogen and progesterone, then the day of the month is also important to know. We saw this graphically in Part I. We'll come back to this shortly.

To address theses factors, three main ways have been developed to measure hormone levels: blood, urine, and saliva. Notice that all three are body fluids. Body fluids are generally never totally isolated from each other. That is, molecules in one body fluid can usually flow into another body fluid. For example, when you eat food, it is mixed with and suspended in saliva, it goes into your stomach, and nutrients then get absorbed into the bloodstream. The blood flows through your body delivering the nutrients, then ultimately through the kidneys, where leftover nutrients and waste products picked up from the body are excreted into the urine. A similar process happens to get rid of wastes through the intestines. In some areas, there is a more defined separation, such as with the blood-brain barrier, in which many toxic molecules in the blood do not easily cross to brain tissue.

BLOOD TESTING

In general, drawing blood is an easy way to get a "snapshot" of a person's hormone levels. The advantages of testing blood include that it is convenient, especially if it can be done while she is in the doctor's office and also does not depend on the person being tested collecting the sample correctly. Disadvantages include that drawing blood is relatively invasive and more painful compared to expelling the fluid into a container, such as with urine or saliva.

Some people assert that blood does not give valid hormone information because hormone levels are always fluctuating in the human body. While it is true that a blood test only measures a moment in time, if the hormone has a long half-life (lasts a long time in the body) then this method still can give a valid measurement. Also, there are quite a few hormones that do have useful, well-established reference ranges on blood tests, such as thyroid function tests. We will come back to the issue of reference ranges. Most importantly, mainstream medicine worldwide has accumulated the most biochemical information on diseases through blood work, and therefore, blood levels are the most common language among doctors. Likewise, most labs will be able to draw hormone blood levels and provide reference ranges for the results. Usually, only specialized labs can run hormone testing on urine and saliva.

URINE TESTING

Measuring hormone levels in the urine is another option. Compared to getting poked with a needle, it is painless to pee in a cup. A single specimen of urine is not considered by most to be a valid measure of hormone levels (although it is useful for many other tests, such as for infection). The best way to use urine to measure hormones is to do what is called a *twenty-four-hour urine collection.*

On one hand, it is easy, but let me clarify how a twenty-four-hour urine collection is done. First, you have to modify caffeine, vitamin, and supplement intake for one or two days before starting. On a day with moderate activity (no exercise) and no alcohol intake, you pick a start time (usually in the morning). For the following twenty-four hours, you pee in a collecting cup (usually bigger than the little cups at the doctor's office) and then pour the urine into a large (half-gallon) collecting container, which might need to be kept in the refrigerator. At the end of the twenty-four hours, you pour some of the urine from the big jug into one or two small vials, which you label and send in to the lab. There are not too many labs that run a comprehensive panel of hormone tests on urine, so you are probably then packaging the urine vials (materials provided by the lab) and sending it by mail to the lab being used.

A big benefit of running a twenty-four-hour urine collection is that you can run a large panel of tests and get a lot of information. The downside is that it is not convenient to do the collection, and even less convenient to repeat the test for follow-up information after treatment. For the purposes of hormone evaluation, this test is usually not covered by insurance. However, there are doctors (especially those with a natu- ropathic orientation) who use this form of testing regularly and with great patient compliance and follow-up.

SALIVA TESTING

Now let's turn to saliva testing. Some people feel that saliva levels of hormones most accurately reflect actual levels of the hormones in the cells of the body. This form of lab testing is not discussed at all in mainstream medical schools, unless it is with derision (the unfortunate human tendency to put down things with which they are unfamiliar).

Saliva testing has the benefit of being non-invasive—again, no needles, just spitting in a container. Again, as with a twenty-four-hour urine collection, producing enough saliva to fill one (or more) little plastic vials is easier said than done. Some saliva kits require only saturating a swab or spot on a card. Again, because most labs do not conduct saliva testing, it is usually necessary to obtain a kit, which has the containers and packaging/shipping materials and instructions. Because this is not a mainstream form of lab testing, most doctors' offices do not stock these kits. They are provided by naturopathic doctors, some alternative pharmacies and through online sources. I think the biggest advantage of saliva testing is that it is convenient to use for hormones that vary throughout the day, particularly adrenal hormones. As with the twenty-four-hour urine collection, most insurances do not cover saliva testing. However, the cost is not usually exorbitant.

REFERENCE RANGES

We have to take a moment to discuss a very important concept in lab testing: the reference range, sometimes erroneously called the "normal range." The usual way to tell if a lab result is normal is to compare it to a range of values. For example, if my kid got an "A" on a test, it's important to know how all the other kids did on the same test. If I learn that all the kids in the class got between an A- and an A+ then my "A" student is actually average in the class, or the test was really easy! The reference range works in the same way—it measures what happens and not necessarily what is *normal* in the group of people being measured. It is calculated by taking the results of a large number of people, putting the results onto a graph and taking the middle ninety-five percent of the results which becomes the reference range (see Figure 3).

Figure 3. How a Lab Reference Range is Determined

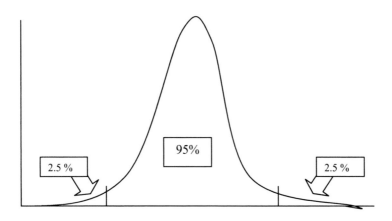

The results form a shape that is compared to a bell-shaped curve. The two outlying ends of the curve are the lab results for, respectively, the top two-and-a-half percent and the bottom two-and-a-half percent of the group that was tested. None of this reference range determination has anything to do with how the people actually feel.

What does this mean in clinical practice? Let's look at what happens if your test result is right above the lower cut-off number of the reference range. First of all, on the lab report, next to that number, there will not be any indication that the result is abnormal. So a doctor or nurse or medical assistant looking over the results quickly will not get flagged to look more carefully at that test result. If that test is measuring a hormone level, it is barely making it into the reference range. Often the reference range is so big that it is easy to see that it is not good to be at the bottom of that large range. For example, "normal" is between 35 and 430, and your level is 36; there really are reference ranges this wide!. In other words, all those people on whom the range is based were not necessarily feeling well—that's just what their test results were. Unfortunately, this is how lab reference ranges are most often used in doctors' practices—people moving quickly are scanning reports for results that are flagged by the lab computer to be outside the reference range. Results that are barely inside the upper or lower limits of the range often get missed.

SPECIFIC HORMONE TESTS

Before we turn to the most commonly used tests to evaluate hormonal status in women, let me backtrack a moment and say that of the following tests we will discuss, most doctors do not in fact run all or most of these tests. We will wrap up this section with tests that are currently gaining in popularity, but are still not in mainstream use by doctors.

FSH

Remember our friend FSH from Menopause 101? Follicle Stimulating Hormone, or FSH, is the most common blood test to assess menopausal status. While it is a useful and important part of a laboratory hormonal evaluation, it is not the final answer as to menopausal status, but rather, has to be put in the context of what is happening with the woman clinically (her symptoms and menstrual cycle).

This hormone is released by the brain in order to stimulate the ovaries to make estrogen, which causes a dominant ovarian follicle cyst to form and begins to prepare the uterine lining for implantation of a fertilized egg. The brain's production of FSH is inhibited by the ovarian hormone *inhibin* which falls as ovarian function declines. So, when inhibin falls (with ovarian aging or surgical removal), FSH rises. We measure FSH on Day 3 of the menstrual cycle to get an idea of ovarian function. If it is nice and low, this generally (not always) means that menopause is *not* imminent. When women in their forties ask me to evaluate their fertility and ability to get pregnant, this is one of the two tests that we run on Day 3 of the menstrual cycle. The other test we run on Day 3 to assess fertility is the *estradiol* level which we will discuss below. If we are not primarily assessing fertility, then FSH and estradiol levels can be checked at any time during the month.

It is possible for stress, and other things that disrupt the menstrual cycle, to cause an increase in the FSH level. This kind of scenario is the unusual case where the FSH level can measure high (over 20 or 30), then be measured again and found to be back in the premenopausal range. In most laboratories an FSH less than 20 indicates that the woman is not fully in menopause. However, as we have already discussed, if she is clinically in the perimenopausal phase (such as with irregular periods) the FSH level does not by itself predict how long this phase will last.

When a woman's periods have been gone for one whole year, an elevated FSH level at this point confirms that ovarian function has dropped down into menopausal levels. Although we can never say never, it would be extremely unlikely after one year with no menstrual periods and an FSH level over 30 for a woman to get pregnant spontaneously. It is only at this point that I am comfortable telling a woman she no longer needs birth control to avoid an unintended pregnancy.

ESTRADIOL

As we discussed in Part I, estrogen occurs in a woman's body in three forms: estrone (E1), estradiol (E2), and estriol (E3). The form most easily and most commonly measured is estradiol. As we have also discussed, the level of estradiol varies throughout the menstrual cycle. The level will also vary during the day to some extent because it may depend on variations in the activity of the estrogen-producing cells during the day. However, the variation during the day is usually minimal. Many tests of E1, E2, and E3 levels can be run on a twenty-four-hour urine collection, with various ratios between them providing additional clinical information.

To pick up on an item mentioned in the previous section, when assessing a woman's fertility we measure estradiol on Day 3 of the cycle. This first half of the menstrual cycle is called the *follicular* phase because, as you recall, the dominant follicle is developing in the ovary during this phase. If the estradiol level is higher than expected this goes along with decreased ovarian function. Let's repeat that: a high estradiol level early in the first half of the cycle means that the ovaries are trying a little too hard. If this is combined with a high FSH level, this indicates *decreased* ovarian function. For the fertility doctors, this makes it less likely that the woman will be able to produce her own egg or eggs to be fertilized for pregnancy, and egg donation is often recommended for better fertility treatment success. Specifically, this would be an FSH over 10 and an estradiol over 70.

In general, because of these fluctuations, measuring estradiol in the blood is not the be-all end-all hormone test in a woman. It can be useful to assess whether there is very low estrogen production versus adequate estrogen production in a woman who is still having some menstrual cycles. It can be run to assess response to estrogen replacement therapy. Ultimately though I rely more on symptomatic response than on what the lab tests say. In other words, if she feels much better but the level did not go up a lot, I do not increase the dose to make the lab result go up. We will get further into this in Step 4, when we discuss treatment options.

PROGESTERONE

As previously mentioned, progesterone is the dominant hormone in the second half of a normal menstrual cycle. Therefore if a woman is having regular twenty-eight-day cycles, we measure the progesterone level in the middle of the second half—Day 21—of her cycle. The part of the menstrual cycle that stays relatively fixed is this second half, between ovulation and the beginning of the menstrual period. This is also called the *secretory* phase of the cycle, in which the endometrial glands secrete mucus and other substances. If a woman's cycle is longer than twenty-eight days then the progesterone measurement must be delayed accordingly. For example, if a woman's cycle is thirty-five days long then the middle of those last two weeks would be Day 28 of her cycle. (You would adjust earlier if her cycle is shorter than twenty-eight days, and measure the progesterone level on Day 18 of a twenty-five-day cycle, for instance.) At this point in the menstrual cycle, if ovulation has occurred properly the progesterone level will be elevated above a value of 3.0 ng/ml on most lab ranges. This level of progesterone in the mid-secretory phase is associated with higher chances of conception and the establishment of a normal pregnancy. For our purposes, a level over 3.0 simply confirms ovulation that month in that cycle in a pre- or perimenopausal woman.

Again, because of the variability of the progesterone levels during a woman's perimenopausal time and in the menopausal transition, it is usually not a firm establisher of menopausal status. It can, however, often give some indication if good ovarian function (ovulation) is continuing and she is still at risk for unintended pregnancy.

TESTOSTERONE

As we discussed in Part I, after the ovaries go through much of the menopausal transition and are no longer ovulating, the last thing they still make is a low level of testosterone. This is what causes women in the menopausal transition, and then in early menopause, to complain sometimes of increased facial hair or acne.

Testosterone is a hormone that most doctors do not routinely test in women. In most doctors' offices, it might be tested if a woman came to a doctor's office with symptoms specifically related to excess testosterone, such as severe acne, excess body hair, or signs of virilization (such as deepening voice).

Testosterone can be measured as *free* testosterone and *total* testosterone. I have seen various combinations of these test results. For example, I have seen a total testosterone in the normal range and a free testosterone that is so low the test cannot measure any! Free testosterone refers to the testosterone molecules that are not bound in the blood to a protein called sex hormone binding globulin (SHBG). Some labs will report the SHBG level because it was measured to calculate the testosterone results. SHBG acts like a sponge and soaks up free testosterone. Estrogen causes an increase in SHBG, which is one way that estrogen produces feminine characteristics (like decreasing body hair). This is also how birth control pills help acne—the estrogen causes an increase in SHBG, which soaks up free testosterone and lowers its acne-producing effect on the skin. Free and total testosterone are useful to measure when your perimenopausal or menopausal concerns include acne, facial or body hair growth, or low sex drive.

DHEA

DHEA stands for dehydroepiandrosterone (phew!). DHEA is secreted by the adrenal glands and is metabolized in the body into estrogen and testosterone. This is important and I want you to keep this in mind. In menopausal women, DHEA from the adrenals results in ninety-five percent of the estrogen activity in their bodies. Most importantly DHEA and its related molecules made by the adrenal glands are responsible for over half of the androgenic activity in all adult women. Because of the testosterone resulting from its metabolism, DHEA. is the major hormone responsible for libido in women.

In comparison with other adrenal hormones, not having enough DHEA is not life-threatening. For example, in people with severe adrenal disease known as Addison's disease when you replace the essential hormone cortisol, they no longer show signs of hormone deficiency. DHEA influences metabolism, seems to influence the immune system, and possibly also has benefits related to cardiovascular disease.

DHEA is easy to measure in the blood and should be measured in the form DHEA *sulfate*. This test can have a very wide reference range. As we discussed above if the lab result on this test is near the bottom of the range, it will often be read as normal. In the anti-aging community of doctors, especially, it is felt that the DHEA sulfate result should be at least in the upper half of the reference range.

OTHER ADDITIONAL TESTS

There are several other important lab tests that can be easily performed with blood work in most laboratories, which I will discuss briefly here.

VITAMIN D

The first and most important additional test that I will discuss here is vitamin D. While most vitamins work by helping other molecular processes happen correctly, in contrast, Vitamin D is a pro-hormone (converted after its production in the skin into the active form) that actually behaves exactly like a hormone. It binds to target cell membranes and causes changes in the function of the cell. There are vitamin D receptors on almost every tissue in the body. The well-known functions of vitamin D include healthy bone metabolism and thyroid function. Research is now pouring in showing benefits to almost every function in the body from optimal levels of vitamin D. An optimal vitamin D level is needed for the immune system, and is associated with lower risk of cancer (including breast cancer), as well as the proper function of many other body systems.

While it is not completely agreed upon what constitutes an optimal level of vitamin D, I will say that in most women in whom I measure vitamin D the results are very low. "Normal" Vitamin D levels always start at about 30 ng/ml, and optimal values are higher, over 50 ng/ml. The main way we get vitamin D is by our skin converting a pre-vitamin D molecule (which comes from cholesterol) into a molecule activated in the kidney into vitamin D. There is very little vitamin D in food, and nowadays, with the widespread use of sunscreen, it is not common to get adequate levels of sun exposure to give adequate levels of vitamin D in the blood. Also, our skin's ability to make vitamin D decreases as we age. This decrease probably begins in our twenties. In other words by the time we are perimenopausal or menopausal our skin's ability to make vitamin D from sunlight is very limited even without sunscreen. In most cases, people need to take vitamin D supplementation in order to have adequate levels of vitamin D. We'll go into detail on amounts of vitamin D supplementation in Step 4.

THYROID TESTING

Many doctors regularly assess thyroid function in women. This is especially commonly tested in women with irregular periods. The problem is that most doctors were taught in medical school to assess thyroid function only by measuring the TSH level. TSH stands for thyroid stimulating hormone. TSH is released from the brain and stimulates the thyroid gland to produce thyroid hormone in two forms referred to as T-3 and T-4 (see Figure 2). A full assessment of thyroid function should include measuring all three of these tests. (There are additional thyroid tests, often measured by endocrinologists, which can be done in addition to this basic panel.) Also, thyroid hormones bind to proteins in the blood as we discussed above with testosterone. Therefore, it important to measure *free* T-3 and *free* T-4 levels; some doctors will also order a *total* T4 to get a full panel on thyroid health.

HIGH-SENSITIVITY C-REACTIVE PROTEIN (HS-CRP)

HS-CRP is another blood test that is growing in popularity. This test is a nonspecific indicator of inflammation in the body. Higher levels of HS-CRP are associated with increased risk for cardiovascular disease. Most anti-aging doctors routinely run this test, and it is starting to gain a foothold in mainstream doctors' offices.

FASTING BLOOD SUGAR

I usually check a fasting blood sugar as part of a general panel of lab work that is called by most labs a comprehensive metabolic panel (CMP). A CMP will check for kidney and liver function, and usually includes a blood glucose level. If this is done with the patient fasting (usually for ten hours) then she will also be screened for prediabetes or diabetes.

CORTISOL

For reasons we have discussed above, I do not routinely measure cortisol levels on my patients. While it is simple to do saliva collection for cortisol levels, it can be inconvenient to collect four samples, the first of which must be very early in the morning, the second two during the day, and the fourth one late at night. More importantly, however, I do not routinely measure cortisol levels because they usually will not change my recommendations. It is usually easy to tell if a person has signs and symptoms of adrenal fatigue without measuring cortisol levels. Also, except under extreme circumstances, medical insurance often will not cover saliva testing and might not even cover cortisol testing in the blood.

It's a general rule we learn in medical school that a test we order is useful if the result will change the recommendations that will be made to the patient. In the case of cortisol and adrenal testing, the results will not change my initial management steps, including improving sleep and diet habits. Saliva cortisol testing can be useful, however, in women who continue to not feel well after initial steps have been taken.

With this information under our belts we are ready to move on to Step 3 - interpreting the results as they apply to you personally in light of the symptoms that we are addressing.

STEP 3

INTERPRET LAB RESULTS IN LIGHT OF SYMPTOMS

In Step 1 you assessed your symptoms. In Step 2 you got thorough lab testing. In order to interpret laboratory results as they apply to you personally, you now need to prioritize your symptoms. I have designed a simple tool, which appears here as a series of questions. This simple "HORMONE QUESTIONNAIRE" appears on the next page, and we will go through each question so you are clear about how to choose your answer of "yes" or "no." Sorting through the many symptoms that we discussed in Step 1 is important to help decide in what order your symptoms should be addressed. As we have discussed, there are basic symptoms related to low female hormone levels and there are symptoms that are more indicative of adrenal or thyroid dysfunction.

To make this tool easy to use with your doctor, you can copy the page, or you can go to http://www.drlizmd.com/DrLizBlog1/dr-lizs-easy-guide-to-menopause/questionnaire and download and print the worksheet which, when filled in and used with the "Treatment Plan Tool," will give you a simple roadmap to work with your doctor to achieve optimal hormone health in perimenopause and menopause.

HORMONE QUESTIONNAIRE

QUESTION 1

Are you menopausal (you've gone one whole year without a menstrual period)?

❑ YES ❑ NO

QUESTION 2

Is your sleep disrupted (you don't get enough sleep, you don't feel refreshed after you sleep, and you don't feel well-rested overall)?

❑ YES ❑ NO

QUESTION 3

Do you suffer from any mood-related symptoms (PMS, crankiness, overly angry or reactive)?

❑ YES ❑ NO

QUESTION 4a

Do you have temperature-related symptoms (hot flashes, night sweats)?

❑ YES ❑ NO

QUESTION 4b

Do you have vaginal dryness, frequent urinary tract infections, or pain with sex?

❑ YES ❑ NO

QUESTION 5

Is your level of sex drive (thoughts about sex and desire for sex) and ability to achieve orgasm less than satisfactory to you?

❑   YES   ❑   NO

QUESTION 6

Do you have unexplained abdominal weight gain?

❑   YES   ❑   NO

QUESTION 7

Do you lack an overall feeling of well-being (energy level, confidence, physical tone, "mojo")?

❑   YES   ❑   NO

QUESTION 8

Have you had general lab work in the past six months (checked vitamin D level, blood sugar, thyroid, and cholesterol panels)?

❑   YES   ❑   NO

QUESTION 1. The first question is to determine whether you are perimenopausal or menopausal. As we said way back in Part I, I use the simplest definition of menopause: one whole year since your last menstrual period (unless you have had your ovaries removed surgically, which officially puts you directly into menopause). I use a very broad definition for perimenopause: you are having menstrual periods that are irregular in any way, and/or you are starting to have hormone-related symptoms described in Step 1. You are in between, in the menopausal transition, if your periods are very irregular and/or your symptoms are very intense and disruptive. Answer "Yes" to this question if you have gone at least one entire year without a menstrual period.

QUESTION 2. This question addresses the quantity and quality of your sleep. My approach with patients is usually to put this up to top priority. A woman who is not sleeping well is inherently more prone to many of the symptoms of the perimenopause and menopause such as mood swings, foggy thinking, irritability, low mood, low sex drive, and weight gain. If fatigue is a major symptom, then you may need even further evaluation of your sleep, such as an overnight study in a sleep lab. In this case it will also be important to evaluate your complete thyroid function. Answer "Yes" if you have any issue in the area of sleep quality.

QUESTION 3. Now we move on to mood relatedquestions. My patients describe to me the following: worsening of their premenstrual syndrome, being short tempered with their partners, co-workers, and children, and generally being more cranky than what the circumstances call for. Some women describe what feels to them like a mild depression; it is important to distinguish these kinds of symptoms from true depression. Answer "Yes" if you have any of the symptoms or concerns listed.

QUESTION 4. This question comes in two parts. The first part addresses symptoms that most women recognize as part of the perimenopause and menopause. This includes symptoms such as hot flashes and night sweats, which are usually due to irregular or low levels of estrogen. The second part of the question relates to lack of estrogen reaching the tissues of the vagina, the urethra, and the base of your bladder. "Pain with sex" refers to pain caused by vaginal dryness and/ or irritation of the vaginal or bladder tissues during intercourse. If you are not sexually active and you feel vaginal dryness, also answer "Yes" to this question.

QUESTION 5. This question is entirely up to your own interpretation of what constitutes a normal sex drive for you. A person who does not have a high desire for sex and does not currently have a sexual partner probably has an appropriate balance for herself in this area at this time. Many of my patients have, for example, husbands who have medical problems with or without erectile dysfunction, and having a low sex drive is not a problem for these women (and in some cases can be helpful). Answer "Yes" if you consider this an area of concern.

QUESTION 6. Weight gain. There's an emotional topic for women. For the purpose of this question, "unexplained" means you are eating moderate amounts of generally healthy foods, you have not changed your exercise level, and you are noticing that your weight is increasing. This weight gain is usually around your midsection (tummy). This includes fat under the skin (that you can pinch) as well as the visceral adiposity (fat around the internal organs) that is associated with health risks. Answer "Yes" to this question if you are experiencing unwanted and unexplained abdominal weight gain.

QUESTION 7. So many women come to me knowing they don't have classic symptoms of menopause such as hot flashes or night sweats, but they say to me things like, "I just don't feel like myself," or

"I feel like I've lost my 'mojo.'" They want to know if this is related to menopause. Well, I believe it is related. You may be trying to work, care for your family, and care for yourself, and your former happy drive to get it all done has left you. So, where you used to feel an energy and accomplishment from your activities, you may now feel anxious and overburdened, and it is not the circumstances that have changed.

You may also feel a lessening of your physical tone (muscle tone), and would typically chalk it up to getting older. The problem is you might be someone who has always exercised regularly, and it is upsetting to see the same exercise activities yielding less physical results on your body.

If you have any of these concerns, answer "Yes" to this question.

QUESTION 8. If you have had general lab work done in the past six months, then it is usually easy to get these results. You can either request them from your primary doctor, or sign a record release in your doctor's office, and everything will be faxed over. If it has been longer than six months, then I recommend you have drawn a full panel of lab work, which will include tests that check kidney and liver function, screen for prediabetes, check your basic blood health, and make sure your cholesterol and other lipids are in a normal range.

I usually give my patient a copy of her lab results, and encourage her to start keeping a file on herself (if she is not doing so already). My patients will often come to see me for an initial consultation with a copy of other lab work ordered by other doctors already in hand. This is very helpful and also helps me avoid turning my patients into pincushions.

Now I am going to go back through the eight questions one more time and discuss how the symptoms connect to the lab tests in the hormone panel.

Question 1. *Follicle-stimulating hormone* (FSH) is often done as the sole determinant of menopausal status. As we've discussed previously the FSH level has to be interpreted in the context of a woman's symptoms. If the FSH is over 20 but she is still having regular periods than she is not clinically in menopause. I have often seen the FSH start to go up (get near or just over 20) in women who are having irregular periods. I do not consider a woman to fully be in menopause until she has had a whole year with no menstrual period regardless of her FSH level.

Question 2. If you are not sleeping well, even though progesterone helps sleep quality (as we will discuss further in Step 4), the progesterone level will not necessarily correlate with your sleep quality. If you are still having menstrual periods, your progesterone level is checked on Day 21 of your cycle (see our discussion in Step 2). This can confirm whether you are ovulating and then making normal amounts of progesterone. As we have discussed previously, progesterone production usually decreases during perimenopause.

Question 3. Mood disturbances can also happen with declining progesterone production. As we just discussed under Question 2, the levels of progesterone on lab tests may not correlate directly with mood-related symptoms (for example, the levels might be normal even though you are suffering from these symptoms).

Question 4. Temperature-related symptoms are first due to fluctuating levels of estrogen then later due to low levels. Therefore, the level of estrogen measured on a blood test will not necessarily correlate with symptoms. In other words, the blood draw might catch the estrogen level when it has spiked up into the normal range. It is initially the ups and downs that give the symptoms, and low levels later on. I have also seen women who do not have temperature symptoms but have vaginal or bladder symptoms; in these situations estrogen levels may be okay but not reaching these tissues. For these reasons, I only check a baseline estradiol level and afterwards only follow symptoms.

Questions 5. DHEA and testosterone levels need to be interpreted in the context of a woman's particular situation. If a woman has a low DHEA level and does not have a current problem with low sex drive I would not necessarily recommend replacing DHEA (or testosterone – see below). By the same token, libido and sexual response often respond to DHEA supplementation. In the case of both DHEA and testosterone, women can often feel an improvement in their energy levels as well as in their overall feeling of well-being with some supplementation of either of these two hormones. This is a very individual discussion to be had between patient and doctor.

Question 6. Regarding abdominal weight gain, DHEA levels may or may not correlate with challenges in this area. As we said earlier, a low DHEA level can often be associated with high cortisol, which is released due to stress, lack of sleep, or high refined carbohydrate intake.

Question 7. Low testosterone level (and low DHEA, since it converts into testosterone) is associated with a lack of vigor, a lack of energy, or a lack of confidence, which in many women can translate into feelings of anxiety. You may also feel poorer physical tone from the same types of exercise. All of this may be related to less testosterone in your system (total testosterone), or less available to your tissues (free testosterone).

Question 8. A general panel of blood tests may include a comprehensive metabolic panel, a complete blood count, a lipid panel, thyroid tests, vitamin D level, and possibly a high-sensitivity C-reactive protein level. See further descriptions of some of these tests back in Step 2.

In Step 3 we have discussed how to prioritize your symptoms and interpret your lab test results in light of these symptoms. Now, we will turn to helping you work with your doctor in a way that will work for you both, so you can get the hormone evaluation that you need, and the support you want at this time in your life. Step 4, let's look at ways to work effectively with your doctor.

TALKING WITH YOUR DOCTOR

Not all doctors are created equal.

The first thing I need to address, in regards to talking with your healthcare providers, is the issue of philosophical differences among doctors. I live between two worlds. On one side is what I call *mainstream* medicine. Others refer to it as conventional medicine. This is the type of medicine in which I was trained (along with most doctors). I was taught to focus on diseases. My job, as I was taught, is to determine the disease that the patient has and to correctly treat it. On my other side is a growing field of medicine is referred to as *anti-aging medicine*, also sometimes called regenerative medicine.

In mainstream medicine, hormone therapy is to be used sparingly. The smallest amounts of hormones necessary to relieve symptoms are to be prescribed for the shortest amount of time possible. In anti-aging medicine, hormones are to be used liberally, often with the goal of achieving the hormone levels of a much younger person.

In my practice, I am often guided by the inclination of my patients in either direction. If she is not comfortable with hormones, then my job is to review the alternatives with her. If I think she would benefit from some form of hormone therapy, I review the evidence with her and often I can reassure her that using hormone therapy to make her feel better during her menopausal transition will usually not be harmful when weighed against the significant benefit that it can bring to her quality of life. If she wants to have full hormone replacement therapy then I am willing and able to do this in partnership with her. If she is somewhere in between, then we work together to determine the optimal hormone replacement that will benefit her quality of life and preserve her health. If she does not want any hormone replacement therapy, we discuss non-hormonal ways to optimize her long-term health.

Because of my emphasis on my patients' *quality of life*, I am far more liberal about hormone replacement therapy than most of my mainstream medicine colleagues. I am not, however, completely won over to the anti-aging side where I also have colleagues whom I respect. In my opinion, not all hormones that decrease with age need to be replaced. In a person who needs several hormones replaced, it is not always necessary to replace them all at once. Hormone replacement can be accomplished in various ways, again with the ultimate goal of improving her quality of life and preserving her health for as long as possible.

Now that we are on the topic of philosophical disagreements among doctors, let's discuss the hot topic of bioidentical hormone therapy.

BIOIDENTICAL HORMONE THERAPY

For the following sections we need to determine some terminology that we can agree upon. One of the reasons many mainstream doctors are not in favor of bioidentical hormone therapy is that the terminology has been bandied about somewhat recklessly up to this point. Allow me to give a little bit of background, as I often review with my patients before they embark on a plan of hormone replacement therapy.

In the United States, we have an interesting system. A great deal of medical research in the US is funded privately by pharmaceutical companies. We have to ask the question: what must happen for a pharmaceutical company to be able to afford to conduct its research? Ultimately, the research must result in a product that can be patented for a number of years and sold through our healthcare delivery system. More specifically (and most typically), the resulting drug must be an effective treatment for a disease or disease symptom. This entire research and development process is closely monitored and regulated by the Food and Drug Administration (FDA). I do not consider this process bad or wrong in any way. It simply is what it is. It is designed a certain way and it proceeds in a certain manner. We live in a society guided by market economy concepts and this model fits well into that context.

So, a pharmaceutical company has to produce a drug—let's call it a new molecule—that can be patented. When a molecule or compound occurs in nature it may not be patented. Take for example honey. You can package honey in different flavors and containers, and you can have your own brand, but you cannot take out a patent on honey. This is at the heart of the issue of bioidentical hormone replacement.

With this issue of what does or does not occur in nature, and therefore what can or cannot be patented, let's look at some terminology.

Natural: Let's start with the term that gets the biggest rise out of mainstream medical doctors. Natural implies "occurring in nature." This term has been used extensively in marketing a wide variety of products (foods as well as drugs). It is assumed by most consumers that "natural" is better than "unnatural." It is important to note that if a hormone or medication has a natural origin, such as from a plant, and has an effect on a symptom or illness, then that product is acting in the same way that any medication acts. Many very strong medications, such as for heart failure and cancer chemotherapy, came originally directly from plants. Therefore, the word "natural" does not necessarily mean having a mild effect. Many product marketers use the word natural to imply proven safety, and this can in fact be a misleading claim. This is why referring to hormones as "natural" irritates many mainstream physicians. We will come back later to the important issue of drug safety.

Synthetic: Now let's look at the term "synthetic." A medication or drug that is synthetic is made in a laboratory. The word "synthetic" literally means "the union of elements to produce compounds." Many drug compounds are originally found in nature; then the active molecule is isolated in a laboratory and created by a "synthetic" laboratory process. The resulting molecule is exactly the same. Some marketing programs have hijacked the term "synthetic" to imply that it is the opposite of "natural"(and therefore bad). In fact, a molecule that is found in nature can sometimes be made more easily in large quantities in a laboratory than it can from gathering large amounts of the original plants from where the molecule came. So, saying that something was made in a laboratory is not to say that it does not occur in nature.

Here is a great example to illustrate these terms and why the debate over terminology is so tricky: Premarin® is an estrogen-replacement product that is actually completely "natural." It is extracted from the urine of pregnant horses (Pre- for pregnant, mar- for mares, -in for urine = Premarin®). It is not synthetic at all! It is not even synthesized in a laboratory; it is entirely from nature, from horses. For doctors who have extra training in bioidentical hormone therapy, the issue is not that this hormone product is not natural, but that it is not similar in any way (is not "bioidentical") to any form of estrogen found in a woman's body.

Pharmaceutically made: This phrase echoes the above mentioned conflicts. Just because something is produced by a pharmaceutical company does not necessarily mean that it is not a molecule that occurs in nature. This phrase has different connotations for different people. For example, most physicians feel that the fact that something is made by a pharmaceutical company means that its development and production was carefully supervised by a well-known set of rules and regulations from the FDA. The resulting product is typically in a precise form, such as a pill, and contains a precise amount of the medication in question, which the patient will then use. In nonmedical circles, this phrase is often intended to have a bad connotation or association with research showing negative effects from the product. As we have discussed, a pharmaceutical company can make a compound ("synthesize" it in a lab) that is exactly like the original that occurs in nature. That is, "pharmaceutically made" can still be "bioidentical."

For example, there is one pharmaceutically made progesterone product that contains the progesterone molecule in the form that it occurs when made by the human body (Prometrium®, which we'll talk about in the next chapter on treatment).

Bioidentical: This term is being used so widely at this point that all affected parties, doctors and their patients, are being drawn together and pushed to agree on what is meant by this term. For a medication or hormone, the term bioidentical means that the molecule in question is the same as the molecule that normally occurs in the human body.

Although many doctors are unfamiliar with or even dismissive of the discussion of bioidentical hormone therapy, to their credit they are beginning to use this particular term correctly. For example, in the mainstream medical literature that I receive, even in articles putting down bioidentical hormone therapy, the term bioidentical is now usually being used correctly.

COMPOUNDED HORMONES

Let me say a word here about compounded hormone products, which are made by compounding pharmacies. Currently, this is a significant topic addressed by major medical organizations, such as the American College of Obstetricians and Gynecologists (ACOG) and the North American Menopause Society (NAMS). Both of these organizations have statements of concern about compounded hormone products. Links to the full statements, and my responses can be found on my Web site at http://www.drlizmd.com/DrLizBlog1/ dr-lizs-easy-guide-to-menopause/statements.

For now, I need to emphasize these important points:

Compounding pharmacies are not unregulated, as pharmaceutical companies and ACOG and NAMS would have us think. There is in fact a different process governing the quality of compounded products than the FDA process that governs drug manufacturing in the United States. All compounding pharmacies are required to meet requirements set by their respective state boards of pharmacy. There is also an organization called the Pharmacy Compounding Accreditation Board (PCAB) which certifies that the pharmacy in question has met a set of stringent criteria for the quality of its personnel, ingredients, and manufacturing facility and equipment. PCAB accreditation is voluntary, and it is easy to determine whether a particular compounding pharmacy has the PCAB Seal of accreditation. Further information on this is available at http://www.drlizmd.com/DrLizBlog1/dr-lizs-easy-guide-to-menopause/pcab. There are two concerns related to scientific evidence: scientific study design and safety.

STUDY DESIGN

The concern over scientific evidence to support individualized therapy is a catch-22. It is true that a large study trying to assess groups of people cannot allow for individual tailoring of a treatment regimen.

If the study allowed this, the results would not be able to be generalized to larger groups. However, it does not make sense to therefore say that it is not appropriate to individualize a woman's hormone replacement therapy regimen. Actually, the ability of a woman to lower the amount of a compounded hormone cream is consistent with the position of both ACOG and NAMS stating that the lowest effective dose of hormones should be used. The issue of scientific studies to assess particular compounded products is challenging because, as we said previously, these products cannot be patented, so the funds for these types of studies will not soon be forthcoming in our current system. Luckily there is extensive data from smaller studies in the United States and from large studies in Europe and Asia confirming the safety and efficacy of various bioidentical hormones.

Also, the discussion of who is and is not a "for-profit" organization is a smokescreen. Literature put out by pharmaceutical companies often emphasizes that ACOG and NAMS are nonprofit organizations (and therefore offer unbiased information) and that information put out by compounding pharmacies is biased because these organizations are for-profit companies. ACOG and NAMS are highly respected organizations that are not oblivious to the business concerns of doctors, and compounding pharmacies are businesses that must provide safe and effective products to people in order to stay in business.

SAFETY

Mainstream medical doctors are justified in being worried about the automatic assumption on the part of the public that anything is 100% safe. As we said before, marketers using the term "natural" often imply this. By the same token, many doctors do not have the time or inclination to become fully familiar with the data regarding all types of hormone replacement therapy. As we said in the last section, there is a great deal of scientific data from around the world (especially Europe and Asia) supporting the efficacy and safety of bioidentical hormone therapy. Second, there is a great deal of important detail in hormone studies done in the United States that could make many doctors more comfortable even with "mainstream" HRT. Many doctors in the US have stopped offering even basic pharmaceutically made HRT options due to fears based on incomplete knowledge.

We will go into more detail about the safety of various treatment options in the next step on treatment options.. For now, suffice it to say that the demand for safe and effective treatments for menopausal symptoms has now joined the increasing demand by patients to be able to discuss a variety of treatment options with their doctors. For women having menopausal symptoms, the days of the doctor simply telling the patient what to do are over.

So let's take Step 4 and get into the details of treatment options.

STEP 4

MAKE A TREATMENT PLAN

Making a Plan to Feel Better—Treatment Options

There are as many different ways to proceed with a treatment plan as there are women in the world. What we can do at this point is use the information and tools that we've discussed so far to help you formulate a plan you can follow to get yourself back to feeling your best. As I keep saying, what we are going for here is your own optimal quality of life.

Remember my patient Anne? After we checked her labs and interpreted the results in light of her individual needs, we embarked on a treatment plan of compounded hormone replacement therapy, and six weeks later she reported the following:

"Now that I am on an individualized hormone therapy program, my weight is under control, I sleep through the night most of the time, I am feeling more energy, my hot flashes during the day are gone (and are mostly gone at night), the acne is minimal, my knees still ache but the other joints are better, and I have an increased interest in sex. I am much happier, and love my sleep. My husband is happier as well!"

Here are the words of one of my patients, Cathy:

When I turned fifty, I was convinced I had lucked out and been one of the few women that never suffered a symptom of menopause. I'd gone to the hilarious play, Menopause—The Musical, about a year earlier and laughed my head off, even though I couldn't relate to most of the jokes. About six months after my birthday, I began experiencing the most extreme night sweats one could only imagine. When my nightly hot flashes started visiting me during the daytime hours, it was more than I could handle. Thankfully, I have naturally curly hair! My personal humidity issue may have been unbearable but my hair looked great! To deal with the intense heat at night, I immediately brought out the fan and attached it to my nightstand so I could have a constant cool wind on my head. My poor dogs and husband...I was burning up and they had frostbite! My husband, (a hospital CEO) had wanted me to see Dr. Lyster but I hesitated because I was convinced she would put me on hormones and I'd gain a ton of weight. Thanks, but no thanks. If given the choice, I'd rather be thin and hotter than hell from suffering gazillion hot flashes a day than be fat and cool as a cucumber. So I suffered for about six to seven months until I couldn't handle it any longer. I shared my concerns with Dr. Lyster during my consult, she ordered some blood work to determine my hormone levels, and she prescribed me some bioidentical hormones in a cream form. Within two days of rubbing the hormone creams into my forearm twice a day, my hot flashes were reduced to one a day and the intensity of the heat was minimal. My sleep had improved 100% and overall, I felt so much better. I think we often don't recognize how shabby we feel until we feel great. And the best part of all: It's been four months and I haven't gained a pound. As a matter of fact, I've lost a few.

As we said earlier, they are many different kinds of hormone replacement therapies. We discussed the several ways that hormone therapy could be administered—by mouth or through the skin. We also discussed a wide variety of symptoms that you may or may not be having and that you may or may not want to use anything to correct.

RISKS VERSUS BENEFITS

I always like to say: life is all about risk versus benefit. Any decision we make in life, especially if it is an important one, involves weighing the risks against the benefits of each choice. Before we get into the steps you will take to develop your own individual plan to feel your best in perimenopause and menopause, let's address the risks of hormone replacement therapy. A complete discussion of this topic could fill a library, so for now I am going to address the two biggest areas of concern for women—breast cancer and cardiovascular disease.

Breast Cancer: Although more women die in the United States from cardiovascular related causes than breast cancer, it is impossible to completely distance oneself from the fear of breast cancer. In my experience, women's biggest concern with hormone replacement therapy is the risk of breast cancer. I can relate to this. I have breasts, and I feel just a little nervousness every time I go for my mammogram, especially since my mom's breast cancer a few years ago.

The media gave tremendous coverage back in 2002 when a large study called the Women's Health Initiative (WHI) stopped one arm (patient group) of the study due to an increase in breast cancer cases. There are a lot of reasons the WHI results should not be generalized to most perimenopausal and menopausal women. The main reasons are that (1) the women in this entire study were in their mid-sixties and were not having menopausal symptoms, (2) they were taking two particular forms of pharmaceutically produced estrogen and progestin, neither of which were bioidentical, and (3) they were taking these hormones by mouth, not through the skin. One highly respected lecturer I heard summed it up as, "Wrong women, wrong hormones, wrong route."

The study arm of the WHI that was stopped was the arm in which women were on combination hormone therapy—that is, they were being given estrogen plus progestin treatment. Remember that a progestin (also called a progestogen) is a laboratory-altered form of progesterone. In some cases, a progestin might be similar to the progesterone molecule and in others it might be similar to the testosterone molecule. The main function of a progestin is to balance the effect of estrogen on the lining of the uterine lining. It often has an even stronger effect than natural progesterone, which allows smaller doses of progestin to be used to control certain aspects of the menstrual cycle. Smaller doses are also used because progestins are also less vulnerable to destruction in the stomach than biologically identical progesterone (we will see shortly how this affects the dosing). Because progestins are not naturally occurring, they have different side effects than bioidentical progesterone.

In these women on estrogen-plus-progestin, an increase was found in their chances of developing breast cancer as compared to the other women in the study (women in the estrogen-only arm and women taking placebos). I want us to look at is the absolute numbers of breast cancer cases in the study. While I would love to share with you lots of information about statistics and how they can be used to prove anything under the sun, that would take us off topic right now. I do need to share with you, however, the statistical concept of *relative risk* as opposed to *absolute* risk. Here are the actual numbers regarding breast cancer in the WHI study: The increase in breast cancer was actually an additional eight women getting breast cancer out of every 10,000 study participants. That is a very small increase in *absolute* risk even though there was an increase in *relative* risk. In fact, I recently read that this increase was not even statistically significant, but it crossed a previously set threshold at which the researchers said they would stop the study (because it was going in a trend towards statistical significance). Doctors disagree about the clinical significance of these numbers. Clinical significance (as opposed to statistical significance) is what the study finding really means to the women affected and the doctors who advise them.

There are two important pieces of information affecting the clinical significance of the study findings that somehow never got broad media coverage. As I mentioned, the WHI study had another arm in which women were only receiving estrogen (these were women who had had a hysterectomy). These women actually had a lower risk of breast cancer than the women taking placebos! All these years later (seven years after the study was first published), the makers of Premarin® are starting to advertise this fact.

The other importance piece of information that I like to emphasize with my patients is that mortality across the board was lower in the women taking hormone therapy (both the estrogen alone and the combination estrogen-progestin groups) than in the women taking placebos. Let's look at this for just a moment. What I'm saying is that even in the group of women who were taking hormones and had the increased number of cases of breast cancer, less of these women died during the study period than the women taking the sugar-pills. The study investigators have not been able to prove why this is the case. Perhaps it is because of the significant decrease in osteoporosis and hip fractures in the women taking hormone therapy. Women who were taking hormone therapy in the study also had less colon cancer. Even in the patients with higher numbers of bad events, such as stroke or heart attack, these were mostly non-fatal events. Again, the mortality in hormone users was lower across the board than in the non-users (placebo group).

Looking particularly at the lower rate of hip fracture in the hormone-users, if you ask the experts in osteoporosis they will emphasize the dramatic adverse impact that a hip fracture can have. There is very high mortality in the first year following a hip fracture for a variety of reasons. It was considered ironic in the medical community that the WH I was the first study to prove that estrogen replacement therapy does, in fact, reduce the risk of hip fracture (ironic because the study results led to so many women stopping their hormones).

Whether or not estrogen causes a new breast cancer is hard to say. We know from studying breast cancer cells that breast cancer tissue can have receptors for both estrogen and progesterone. It is likely that the original event of a breast tissue cell turning into a cancer cell and then growing into a tumor is not caused by estrogen. At the same time, it is also likely, especially in an estrogen receptor-positive breast cancer, that estrogen helps breast cancer cells grow. Because of this, factors such as personal and family medical history will affect decisions on hormone replacement therapy.

Luckily our knowledge is growing and will only continue to grow to be able to assess in detail a woman's risk for developing breast cancer. For example, we are currently seeing a big increase in genetic testing both for gene mutations that lead to breast and ovarian cancers as well as genetic testing of breast cancer tissue itself to improve cancer treatment.

Cardiovascular Disease: Let's turn our attention briefly to the huge topic of cardiovascular disease in women. As I mentioned earlier, this is by far the biggest cause of death in women in the United States. (The number one cause of death is heart disease and number two is stroke, and these are both in the category of cardiovascular disease.) When estrogen therapy became very popular in the 1970s, it was observed that women taking hormone therapy had less cardiovascular disease. In fact, this is why the manufacturer of Premarin and Provera undertook the WHI study—in order to prove that hormone replacement therapy prevents cardiovascular disease.

Since the first WHI findings were published in 2002, it has now become clear that the age at which a woman starts hormone therapy is crucial. Recall that the women in the WHI hormone group were in their sixties, and had no menopausal symptoms. They had an increase in cardiovascular events but not in mortality from these events. It seems that a woman's body that has low hormone levels and no related symptoms has adapted to the low hormone levels. If hormones are then given, it can cause problems, as was seen in the study.

Results from this study are still being analyzed, and additional conclusions related to the risks of the hormones used are still being released by the researchers of the WHI. Unfortunately, the media and many doctors continue to generalize these results to all hormone therapy and all menopausal women, despite the study's pitfalls we have discussed.

Many smaller studies (both in the United States and abroad) have shown important benefits from estrogen. It is well documented that estrogen has a beneficial effect on blood lipids. It raises the HDL ("good" cholesterol) and lowers LDL ("bad" cholesterol). Estrogen directly affects and improves the function of the cells that line the blood vessels of the body. Under the influence of estrogen, these cells (endothelial cells) resist the formation of plaque (atherosclerosis). If a woman's cells have not been exposed to estrogen for a long period of time, such as the women in their sixties in the WHI study, the number and activity of estrogen receptors in their blood vessels decrease. In these women, proceeding to give estrogen can actually result in a harmful inflammatory response. This is exactly what was demonstrated in the WHI study—women who had not been on hormones for many years were given hormones, and then had adverse events. Many studies show that women get a benefit from hormone therapy given within five years of going into menopause; there seems to be a "window of opportunity" in which hormone therapy does give women cardiovascular protection.

In this brief treatment of a very extensive topic, a last important topic is the incidence of Type 2 Diabetes in menopausal women. The WHI study showed that women in both groups (estrogen only and estrogen-progestin therapy) had reduced incidence of new-onset diabetes. They had less insulin resistance, better lipid levels, and lower blood pressure. The women without diabetes had less abdominal obesity, and the women with diabetes had lower fasting blood sugar levels. The conclusion for now is that the blood vessel benefits of HRT that help the heart, also help the blood vessel complications related to diabetes.

CREATING A TREATMENT PLAN

Earlier, I talked about weighing risks versus benefits. Because the above discussion can be so time-consuming for doctors in the office, it will help you work effectively with your doctor to have this knowledge and to know your options. Now that I've given you a brief overview of the currently known risks and benefits of hormone therapy, let's now turn to the specific benefits that you can receive from specific hormone treatments.

Your first step in developing a treatment plan is to determine what symptom is the most disruptive for you. At this point you have already used the questionnaire provided to assess your symptoms. If disrupted sleep is on your list of symptoms and was not at the top of your list before you answered the eight questions, I am now asking you to move that up to a top priority. It is difficult if not impossible to achieve hormone balance and a healthy without adequate quantity and quality of sleep.

Let's take our prior discussion of philosophy and apply it directly to the issue of hormone therapy. As I said before, in the mainstream medical community hormone replacement therapy is to be used in the least amount for the least time possible. As the data from the 2002 Women's Health Initiative (WHI) study continues to be analyzed, it is beginning to become clear that it is actually less risky to begin hormone therapyduring the menopausal transition or early in menopause rather than later on, after symptoms have gone away.

The easiest women to work with for an optimal hormone replacement therapy program are women who meet the definition of menopause, that is to say they have not had a period for at least one full year. If this is the case for you then you are like a blank canvas and you can work with your doctor to paint a beautiful picture of menopausal vigor and health. If this is not the case for you, then I ask you to be patient and willing to work with your doctor over a period of time to get your best results from HRT.

Why is symptom relief more difficult if a woman is not all the way in menopause? If a woman is not completely through her menopausal transition, her ovaries may still be making some estrogen. This may be leading to estrogen excess symptoms such as breast tenderness and headaches. In this situation, progesterone treatment will be helpful. It can be hard to determine whether to give the progesterone treatment in a way that imitates the cycle (for example, to give the progesterone the second half of each month) or to give the progesterone therapy on a daily basis. This can be difficult because the menstrual cycles might be so irregular that we don't have a regular "Day 1" of the cycle on which to start counting each month. Also, bleeding may be irregular due to erratic ovarian hormone production during this time. Again, you have to be willing to work with your doctor, as it may take a little longer to get your symptoms settled.

Also, in younger women symptoms usually tend to be more intense. If you choose not to take any HRT, in the vast majority of cases symptoms will decrease over time and will eventually go away. There can be, however, some women whose symptoms never completely resolve. Studies show that symptoms can typically last as long as eight years (and I have seen longer) if not treated.

As I always say to my patients, the main issue overall is quality of life. It is not necessary (and even unhealthy) to feel terrible. Everything in life is "risks versus benefits." If your symptoms are severe and disruptive and clearing them up would have huge benefits, then in most cases, this benefit would outweigh the risks of hormone replacement therapy.

Now I am going to take you through the "Treatment Plan Tool" on the next page. You will see that it is organized to match the hormone questionnaire that you have already filled in. That questionnaire had eight questions that you answered. The tool on the next page is organized into eight "answers." I put this in quotation marks because I am not the kind of doctor who ever states that she has the final answer for her patients. How you proceed is ultimately based on your own understanding of your body and your choices. This tool is also not meant to replace your own consultation with your doctor (or doctors, if you have any medical problems). It is meant to be a guide to help you understand how you can individualize your hormone therapy to feel your best. After we go through the tool, I will take you through a summary of each treatment choice category.

TREATMENT PLAN TOOL

"ANSWER" 1

If you have not gone one whole year without a menstrual period than you need to <u>consider whether you may need birth control</u> along with symptom relief.

"ANSWER" 2

If you have any degree of sleep disruption, or if fatigue is an important problem to you, then consider <u>bioidentical progesterone</u> as part of your program. If you are still having menstrual periods, then you may need the progesterone ten to fourteen days per month rather than everyday.

"ANSWER" 3

Mood-related symptoms will often respond to <u>bioidentical progesterone.</u> Also, low-dose birth control pills (even if you do not need birth control) can help stabilize mood.

"ANSWER" 4a

Temperature-related symptoms respond to <u>estrogen</u> therapy (usually a daily regimen). Mild symptoms may respond to <u>DHEA</u> (especially if your DHEA level is low). There are also <u>non-hormonal</u> treatment options.

"ANSWER" 4b

Vaginal and bladder symptoms respond best to <u>topical estrogen</u> (daily at first, then less). There are some <u>non-hormonal</u> options.

"ANSWER" 5

Daily <u>DHEA</u> replacement is often helpful with sexual function; it usually takes four to six weeks to take effect. Also, <u>testosterone</u> therapy may be helpful.

"ANSWER" 6

DHEA, nutrition, and physical activity are the main factors in abdominal weight gain (after medical problems are ruled out).

"ANSWER" 7

Overall feeling of well-being, libido, and physical tone are helped by DHEA and testosterone.

"ANSWER" 8

While hormone therapy may help certain medical problems, you also need to get the right evaluation and treatment for such problems. You also need an optimal vitamin D level for good health. The latest recommendation for Vitamin D dosing is 5,000 iu daily.

In the Treatment Plan Tool, we brought up the following categories of hormone therapy:

1)   Birth control

2)   Progesterone

3)   Estrogen

4)   DHEA

5)   Testosterone

Let's take these categories one at a time. A summary in chart form will follow, and will include common doses and the equivalents for compounded products to pharmaceutically made products.

1) Birth control: There are two options in this category that can help with perimenopausal symptoms as well as provide effective birth control. Either of these options may be appropriate in a woman with irregular bleeding after it has been determined that there is no other cause of the bleeding that needs other treatment.

a. First, low-dose birth control pills (BCPs) can be a way to address several perimenopausal concerns at once. In women who have not yet gone one full year without a menstrual period, BCPs will regulate the period and provide protection against unplanned pregnancy at the same time. After women in their teens and early twenties, women in their late forties are the next largest group in which unintended pregnancy occurs. If you are having some hot flashes or night sweats, BCPs will also relieve this. BCPs are NOT a good option for women over thirty-five years of age who are current smokers, due to the increased risks of cardiovascular problems such as heart attack, stroke, or systemic blood clots.

b. The second option in this category is the levonorgestrel-releasing intrauterine system (known by the trade name Mirena®). This is an intrauterine device that releases very small amounts of a progestin into the lining of the uterus, making the lining very thin, which in turn makes menstrual bleeding very light. It was just approved in October of 2009 by the FDA for the indication of treating heavy menstrual bleeding (it was previously officially only approved for birth control). It also provides highly effective birth control, partly because it does not depend on the woman using it having to remember to do anything like taking a pill every day. The Mirena® device is inserted by a doctor (or nurse practitioner or physician's assistant) in the office, and is approved in the US to stay in place for up to five years (in other countries it is approved for seven years) providing excellent birth control and control of irregular bleeding. An additional advantage of the Mirena® is that the progestin it releases into the uterine lining has been proven to be enough to protect the endometrium from the stimulating effects of estrogen.

2) **Progesterone:** Bioidentical progesterone (as distinct from a progestin) is available three main ways.

    a. First, it is available over-the-counter in low-dose cream formulations. These formulations usually have about twelve to twenty milligrams (mg) of progesterone per gram of cream. The production of these creams is private, with the exact composition not disclosed (called "proprietary") and the manufacture is not regulated either by the FDA or by any pharmacy authority. I have personally observed, however, good efficacy for help with mood and sleep quality in my patients.

    b. Second, it is available as a compounded product: a cream, capsule, or sublingual form (also called a troche ["tro-key"]). Compounding pharmacies that make these products in large quantity are able to charge less for the product. In many cases, insurances will cover these products (that is determined on an individual basis).

c. Third, there is one pharmaceutically made bioidentical progesterone product called Prometrium®; this form is called micronized progesterone. This product has been tested extensively and shown to have the benefits of other progestins regarding protecting the endometrium in women taking estrogen replacement therapy. The 1996 study called the PEPI (Postmenopausal Estrogen/Progestin Interventions) trial gave this bioidentical product equal footing with other pharmaceutical progestins used in mainstream medicine. The sedating effect on the brain of bioidentical progesterone only happens about ten percent of the time with Prometrium® as opposed to most of the time with compounded progesterone products (progesterone molecules preferentially concentrate in brain cells, which gives the calming effect and some research also shows protection of brain cells against injury).

3) Estrogen: If at all possible, the preferred route of administration of any kind of estrogen therapy is *through the skin* or mucous membranes, rather than by mouth. The scientific data supporting this has been accumulating now for several decades, and supportive articles are now appearing regularly in my mainstream medical publications. (Also see http://www.drlizmd.com/DrLizBlog1/dr-lizs-easy-guide-to-menopause/references.) These articles show that oral estrogen has the "first-pass" effect on the liver, where the estrogen concentrates in the liver and stimulates the production of the clotting factors made there, which then promotes the formation of blood clots in the body significantly more often than when the estrogen is applied to the body through the skin. By "through the skin," there are several options.

a. Transdermal is most commonly in the form of patches that are applied to the abdomen or hips, or cream/gel/sprays applied to areas of skin, such as the arms (the inner arms have thin skin and blood vessels just underneath) or the abdomen, hips or thighs.

b. Other forms of "through the skin" include: *Sublingual*, which is made in a compounding pharmacy and goes through the thin mucous membranes under the tongue (the hard part is avoiding swallowing the hormone preparation). Another is *Transmucosal*, which is made either pharmaceutically or in a compounding pharmacy, and is administered through other mucous membranes, such as the vaginal epithelium (skin) or through the skin of the labia. *Subcutaneous*—made by specialized companies—consists of pellets of estradiol that are inserted under the skin; while they are often effective and deliver steady levels of hormone for several months, the pellet cannot be removed if the dose is not right for you.

Note: I will also make special mention at this point of a compounded product called Biest (listed below in the chart). We have been talking a lot about estradiol. If you recall back to Part I, we talked about how estrogen occurs in a woman's body in three forms: estrone, estradiol, and estriol. Since the goal of a compounded product is to copy nature, compounded estrogen was first made as "Tri-est," with a composition imitating the proportions of each of these three estrogen forms in the female body. Research later showed that because of the normal conversion between these three forms, it was only necessary to make "Bi-est," containing estradiol and estriol (as these two forms metabolize into the right proportion of estrone). There is a heated controversy still going on over estriol. Here is the bottom line: while the

FDA does not officially approve estriol, there is a huge amount of scientific data supporting the safety and efficacy of estriol and estriol-containing products. You can find more about this at http://www.drlizmd. com/DrLizBlog1/dr-lizs-easy-guide-to-menopause/estriol.

4) **DHEA:** This hormone, as previously mentioned, is available in over-the-counter tablet or capsule form, or it can be put into compounded products (oral or transdermal). In most published studies of this adrenal hormone, the DHEA was given orally; this is the most commonly used form. Because it is over-the-counter, DHEA is available in many brands and formulations. It is manufactured and distributed in the US as a food and not a drug, so while many scientific studies support the safety and efficacy of DHEA, this information is not presented in conventional medical training and therefore DHEA is not widely recommended at this time by mainstream doctors.

5) **Testosterone:** Testosterone is a controlled substance in the United States (only available by prescription from a licensed doctor). Women can get the beneficial effects of testosterone as a metabolic byproduct of DHEA. More commonly, it is provided through the skin in a compounded cream or orally in a capsule. It is also available as a subcutaneous (under the skin) pellet. There was one pharmaceutically made product containing a non-bioidentical form of testosterone, but it was very recently taken off the market (according to the manufacturer it was for business, not safety reasons).

In some cases, women will get a better response depending on the route of administration of the hormone. For example, while most women get very good results from transdermal hormone replacement therapy (which I have recommended as the preferred route), there are individuals who respond better to taking the hormones by mouth. As I keep saying, the goal is improved quality of life, and if the benefits outweigh the risks, then we are on a good path.

A BRIEF WORD ABOUT NON-HORMONAL TREATMENTS

You are probably aware of many herbal and other types of non-hormonal treatments that are on the market for menopausal symptoms. A complete discussion of herbal therapies is outside the scope of this book and, luckily, there are many books on the subject. This is of special concern to breast cancer survivors, or women who have had other medical problems in the past, such as certain other cancers, stroke or heart attack, or blood clots, who are not considered by most doctors to be good candidates for hormonal therapy,

One important and common example is the treatment of severe vaginal dryness in breast cancer survivors. If you are in this group, there are many good water-based lubricants and vaginal moisturizers that may provide enough relief for you. The issue of increased bladder infections might be harder to resolve than the issue of comfort during sex. While the risk versus benefit is to be determined between you and your doctor, most of our knowledge supports the use of local topical estrogen treatment for a limited time, because it does not enter the bloodstream through thin tissue in significant amounts (the thin tissue has less blood flow through it). However, you will not be seeing this in mainstream medical publications just yet as an official recommendation. Scientific data actually shows that estriol, a weaker estrogen than estradiol, has a lot of receptors in vaginal tissue, and might even be protective of breast cells. Hopefully, the politics will settle down and more research and testing will confirm the option of vaginal estriol in breast cancer survivors. But don't forget, if it can't be patented, the research won't be coming any time soon, at least in our current system.

When considering all treatment options, and when hearing warnings about certain treatments, remember to learn the absolute risk, and not look only at the relative risk. If something "doubles the risk" but that means it goes from two out of 100,000 to four out of 100,000, you might still be willing to take a chance that you'll be among the 999,996 who are fine. Above all, remember to compare the possible risks with the possible benefits. In this way, you and your doctor can make an informed decision that will maximize your quality of life.

Below is a summary of common dosages and dosage ranges of the most common bioidentical and pharmaceutically made hormone replacement products. This is not an exhaustive list; it is only meant to help you and your doctor recognize the most common names and dosages of hormone compounds. Your actual treatment should be tailored to your own needs and your individual response to hormone therapy.

Last, but not least, we will talk about what your personal follow-up plan will look like. Let's move on to Step 5, our final step, which provides tools on how to stick to your health and wellness strategies.

Hormone	Routes of Administration	Common HRT Daily Dosing	Pharmaceutical Product Name and/ or Dose Equivalent	Dose Range	Common Timing Of Dose
Birth Control Pills	Oral	20mcg ethinylestradiol* Various	N/A	20 - 35 mcg ethinylestradiol*	Daily, same time (Not for women over 35 who smoke)
Bioidentical **Progesterone**	Oral:compounded Oral: Prometrium* Transdermal (compounded)	100mg 100 or 200 100mg	As stated for Prometrium*	100-200mg 100-400mg 20-100mg	Bedtime (Usual dose is less than 100mg for women with no uterus who need progesterone)
Estrogen	Oral:Estradiol* Transdermal: • Compounded (Biest) • Patch E2 • Spray E2 • Gel	.05 mg 2.5 mg/g 0.5 mg/day 2 sprays	Estrace* 0.5 mg Premarin* 0.625 mg Vivelle Dot* Climara* Evamist* Elestrin*	0.5 - 1 0.3 - 1.25 mg 1.25-5mg (or more) 0.025 - 0.1 mg 1 to 3 sprays	Daily Daily Twice weekly Daily
DHEA	Oral (OTC) Compounded (oral or transdermal)	10 mg 10 mg		5 to 25 mg 5 to 25 mg (or more)	Daily (AM) May further increase dose if no side effects
Testosterone	Oral or transdermal (compounded)	1.25 mg		1.25-2.5 mg	Daily

103

Step 5

FOLLOW-UP AND MAINTENANCE

As I have said before, if you are completely in menopause then it will be relatively easy for you and your doctor to work together and follow the steps we've gone through to layout a plan for your hormonal health and well-being at this time in your life. If you are perimenopausal, please be patient and work in partnership with your doctor until you are feeling well hormonally. Now we're going to turn to the issue of the timing of your appointments with your doctor.

HOW LONG WILL IT TAKE
UNTIL I FEEL BETTER?

After your initial consultation, and then your review of lab work, follow-up appointments with your doctor will depend on a few things. Most importantly it depends on the severity of your symptoms and which symptoms we are addressing first. For example, if your main issue is hot flashes and night sweats, we can tell pretty quickly whether the prescribed hormone therapy is helping—usually within two weeks. If your main issue is lack of libido, we have to allow more time to see if hormone therapy is helping—at least four to six weeks.

When you are having lab work done to assess your hormone levels, I am perfectly comfortable with you starting your hormone therapy right after the blood is drawn (or the urine or saliva collected). Some women are more comfortable waiting to start hormone therapy until after they come in to see me to discuss the results. This is fine if your symptoms are not severe, or if your symptoms could be explained better by waiting for the results (such as mood changes, irritability, or fatigue).

If your main issue is temperature-related—symptoms such as hot flashes and night sweats—you can usually expect these symptoms to start to improve with estrogen therapy after only a few days. If you do not have an improvement in these symptoms after taking estrogen replacement for two weeks then you should talk with your doctor about possibly increasing the dose.

If your main symptom is disrupted sleep and you are not having temperature-related symptoms that you are aware of then it can take progesterone therapy as little as a few nights or as long as two to four weeks to make a difference for you.

If you are using DHEA for issues such as low libido or low energy level, then it is reasonable to give it four to six weeks before you decide if it is making a difference. Remember, DHEA is working with your body's wisdom and converting into estrogen and testosterone in a balance that is unique to you. I would also give testosterone replacement therapy a four to six-week time frame in order to evaluate if it is making any difference in how you feel.

Overall, I usually determine the first follow-up visit based on the severity of my patient's symptoms. The soonest follow-up that I typically do in the office is four weeks. If her symptoms are not severe, a more typical follow-up visit will usually be at about eight weeks from when she starts her hormone replacement therapy.

After this first follow-up visit, it depends on the individual woman's scenario. If we needed to do any adjustments of the hormone type or dose, then I would again follow-up at six to eight weeks.

If she responded well to the initially prescribed doses of hormones and she does not feel that she would like to check in with me again quickly, a typical next follow-up visit would be three months later

At the follow-up visit I try to learn about her total experience with HRT so far. I like to know if she had good service at her pharmacy, if her prescriptions were affordable, and in what form did the pharmacist dispense her hormone therapy. For example, if I prescribed hormone creams, I'd like to know in what dispenser form my patient received her cream, whether it is in a syringe (no needle!), in a jar, or in a pump. This is essential information for me to be able to offer any phone advice or follow-up, especially if she is having any confusion regarding the dosing. While I am thinking in terms of milligrams of hormones, my patients is thinking in terms of amount of cream so I need to be able to know how she is measuring out the cream. Several pharmaceutically made estrogen creams, gels, and sprays come in particular dispensers according to the brand.

I only do follow-up blood testing if she is supplementing anything that had a very low level on initial lab work, such as DHEA or vitamin D levels. I also may do follow-up blood work if she is not responding to any part of the hormone therapy. In other words, I do not do the follow-up blood work on a set schedule; it is tailored to my patient's individual needs. If a follow-up blood level is low but my patient's symptoms have resolved, I usually will not change any dose of anything. I am treating my patient, and not the lab test result. For example, if the estrogen therapy has completely cleared up her hot flashes, but the blood level is still low (or the progesterone treatment is helping her sleep like a baby but the blood level is low), I don't change a thing. Her quality of life is improving and that is our goal.

If all is well, and I am seeing her a whole year after starting her HRT, we may check levels of hormones to know what are her current levels for comparison during the coming year (in case anything changes). On rare occasion, I have asked an enthusiastic patient or two to scale back on vitamin D, if her level was over 100 ng/ml, although it is unlikely that she was headed for major toxicity. Often, this yearly recheck of labs will include general labs (cholesterol, metabolic, and thyroid panels) if they were not checked elsewhere during the year.

My grandma used to say (I am translating from the Spanish), "The years do not come alone." Once your uncomfortable perimeno-pausal and menopausal symptoms resolve, you have to do your part in staying as healthy and strong as you can. You must address all the areas around the "circle of health" in order to truly maintain hormonal balance and good health.

Part III

THE BIG PICTURE

ARE HORMONES ALL YOU NEED TO FEEL BETTER?

No! Although we have spent time focusing on the medical area of the circle of health— hormones and hormone balance—no woman's life is completely balanced without the other areas of the circle. Each of us must have the right amounts of the right foods, the right amounts of the right kinds of exercise, as well as spiritual well-being and mental fulfillment. Not to mention enough sleep! Excess fat tissue is hormonally disruptive, and there is no time like the present to do the work necessary to shed excess fat and the health risks it carries. As Barbara Sher, author and life coach, says in her book title *"It's Only Too Late If You Don't Start Now!"*

A very well-known and highly respected menopause and hormone expert in the world of mainstream medicine, Dr. Wulf Utian, was asked in an interview, "How long is it safe to take hormone therapy?" His answer was my favorite answer yet: "From one annual exam to the next." Every woman can take things one year at a time during perimenopause and menopause, and meet the challenges in partnership with her doctor. I wish for every woman to have a doctor she can trust and talk openly with, and with whom she can create and follow her own path to optimal hormone health.

At this point, I hope that you have gained a few things. First, I hope you have gained useful information to help you know that if you are having menopause-related symptoms, you are not going crazy! Second, I hope that you have developed a way to address your symptoms in a step-by-step manner in order to be able to feel your best. Third, I hope you can use this information to work with your doctor to implement your plan. Last, and perhaps most of all, I hope you feel empowered to make the second half of your life your best.

APPENDIX A

QUESTION 1

Are you menopausal (you've gone one whole year without a menstrual period)?

☐ YES   ☐ NO

QUESTION 2

Is your sleep disrupted (you don't get enough sleep, you don't feel refreshed after you sleep, and you don't feel well-rested overall)?

☐ YES   ☐ NO

QUESTION 3

Do you suffer from any mood-related symptoms (PMS, crankiness, overly angry or reactive)?

☐ YES   ☐ NO

QUESTION 4a

Do you have temperature-related symptoms (hot flashes, night sweats)?

☐ YES   ☐ NO

QUESTION 4b

Do you have vaginal dryness, frequent urinary tract infections, or pain with sex?

❑ YES   ❑ NO

QUESTION 5

Is your level of sex drive (thoughts about sex and desire for sex) and ability to achieve orgasm less than satisfactory to you?

❑ YES   ❑ NO

QUESTION 6

Do you have unexplained abdominal weight gain?

❑ YES   ❑ NO

QUESTION 7

Do you lack an overall feeling of well-being (energy level, confidence, physical tone, "mojo")?

❑ YES   ❑ NO

QUESTION 8

Have you had general lab work in the past six months (checked vitamin D level, blood sugar, thyroid, and cholesterol panels)?

❑ YES   ❑ NO

TREATMENT PLAN TOOL

"ANSWER" 1

If you have not gone one whole year without a menstrual period than you need to <u>consider whether you may need birth control</u> along with symptom relief.

"ANSWER" 2

If you have any degree of sleep disruption, or if fatigue is an important problem to you, then consider <u>bioidentical progesterone</u> as part of your program. If you are still having menstrual periods, then you may need the progesterone ten to fourteen days per month rather than everyday.

"ANSWER" 3

Mood-related symptoms will often respond to <u>bioidentical progesterone.</u> Also, low-dose birth control pills (even if you do not need birth control) can help stabilize mood.

"ANSWER" 4a

Temperature-related symptoms respond to <u>estrogen</u> therapy (usually a daily regimen). Mild symptoms may respond to <u>DHEA</u> (especially if your DHEA level is low). There are also <u>non-hormonal</u> treatment options.

"ANSWER" 4b

Vaginal and bladder symptoms respond best to topical estrogen (daily at first, then less). There are some non-hormonal options.

"ANSWER" 5

Daily DHEA replacement is often helpful with sexual function; it usually takes four to six weeks to take effect. Also, testosterone therapy may be helpful.

"ANSWER" 6

DHEA, nutrition, and physical activity are the main factors in abdominal weight gain (after medical problems are ruled out).

"ANSWER" 7

Overall feeling of well-being, libido, and physical tone are helped by DHEA and testosterone.

"ANSWER" 8

While hormone therapy may help certain medical problems, you also need to get the right evaluation and treatment for such problems. You also need an optimal vitamin D level for good health. INDEX*

INDEX

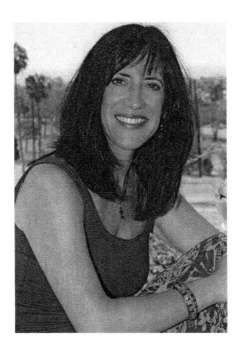

With over 15 years experience as an OB/GYN, Doctor Liz helps women balance hormones, reach and maintain a healthy weight, and regain wellness in their lives. She graduated with honors from Cornell University, completed medical school at the University of California at Irvine , and earned her Master of Public Health degree at UCLA in Health Education. Doctor Liz is in private practice in Orange County, California and is a wife and a mom of two active boys. Doctor Liz can be reached via her Web site www.DrLizMD.com.

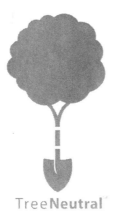

TreeNeutral

Advantage Media Group is proud to be a part of the Tree Neutral™ program. Tree Neutral offsets the number of trees consumed in the production and printing of this book by taking proactive steps such as planting trees in direct proportion to the number of trees used to print books. To learn more about Tree Neutral, please visit **www.treeneutral. com.** To learn more about Advantage Media Group's commitment to being a responsible steward of the environment, please visit **www. advantagefamily.com/green**

Easy Guide To Menopause is available in bulk quantities at special discounts for corporate, institutional, and educational purposes. To learn more about the special programs Advantage Media Group offers, please visit **www. KaizenUniversity.com** or call 1.866.775.1696.

Advantage Media Group is a leading publisher of business, motivation, and self-help authors. Do you have a manuscript or book idea that you would like to have considered for publication? Please visit **www.amgbook.com**